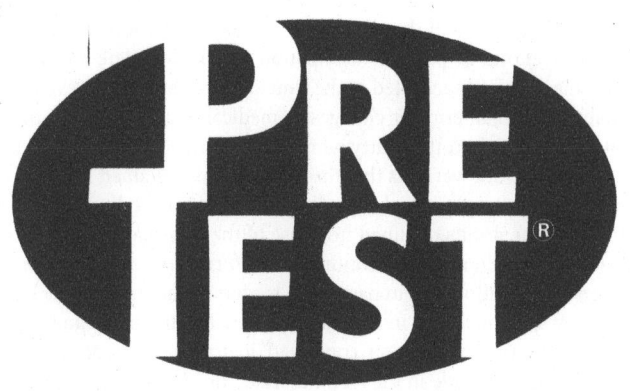

Chest Radiology
PreTest® Self-Assessment and Review

NOTICE

Medicine is an ever-changing science. As new research and clinical experience broaden our knowledge, changes in treatment and drug therapy are required. The authors and the publisher of this work have checked with sources believed to be reliable in their efforts to provide information that is complete and generally in accord with the standards accepted at the time of publication. However, in view of the possibility of human error or changes in medical sciences, neither the authors nor the publisher nor any other party who has been involved in the preparation or publication of this work warrants that the information contained herein is in every respect accurate or complete, and they disclaim all responsibility for any errors or omissions or for the results obtained from use of the information contained in this work. Readers are encouraged to confirm the information contained herein with other sources. For example and in particular, readers are advised to check the product information sheet included in the package of each drug they plan to administer to be certain that the information contained in this work is accurate and that changes have not been made in the recommended dose or in the contraindications for administration. This recommendation is of particular importance in connection with new or infrequently used drugs.

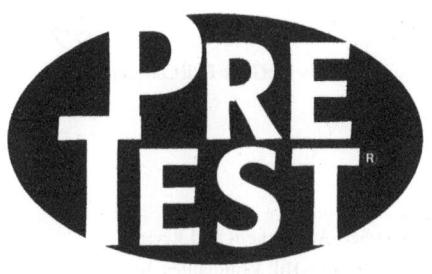

Chest Radiology

PreTest® Self-Assessment and Review

JUZAR ALI, M.D., FRCP(C)
Associate Professor of Clinical Medicine
Louisiana State University Health Sciences Center
School of Medicine in New Orleans
Section of Pulmonary/Critical Care Medicine
New Orleans, Louisiana

WARREN R. SUMMER, M.D.
Howard A. Buechner Professor and Section Chief,
Pulmonary & Critical Care Medicine
Louisiana State University Health Sciences Center
School of Medicine in New Orleans
Director, Pulmonary Services
Medical Center of Louisiana at New Orleans
Chief, Pulmonary Services
Ochsner Clinic
New Orleans, Louisiana

McGraw-Hill
Medical Publishing Division
PreTest® Series

New York   Chicago   San Francisco   Lisbon
London   Madrid   Mexico City   Milan
New Delhi   San Juan   Seoul
Singapore   Sydney   Toronto

McGraw-Hill

A Division of The **McGraw·Hill** Companies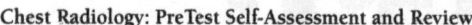

Chest Radiology: PreTest Self-Assessment and Review

Copyright © 2001 by the **McGraw-Hill Companies,** Inc. All rights reserved. Printed in the United States of America. Except as permitted under the United States Copyright Act of 1976, no part of this publication may be reproduced or distributed in any form or by any means, or stored in a data base or retrieval system, without the prior written permission of the publisher.

1 2 3 4 5 6 7 8 9 0 DOC/DOC 0 9 8 7 6 5 4 3 2 1

ISBN 0-07-135959-1

This book was set in Berkeley by North Market Street Graphics.
The editor was Catherine Johnson.
The production supervisor was Lisa Mendez.
Project management was provided by North Market Street Graphics.
The text designer was Jim Sullivan / RepoCat Graphics & Editorial Services.
The cover designer was Li Chen Chang / Pinpoint.

This book is printed on acid-free paper.

Library of Congress Cataloging-in-Publication Data

Ali, Juzar.
    Clinical chest radiology : PreTest self-assessment and review : chest X-ray interpretation with clinical stems and review / Juzar Ali, Warren R. Summer.
    p. ; cm.
    Includes bibliographical references and index.
    ISBN 0-07-135959-1 (pbk.)
    1. Chest—Radiography—Examinations, questions, etc.
    2. Chest—Diseases—Diagnosis—Examinations, questions, etc.
    3. Diagnosis, Radioscopic—Examinations, questions, etc.
    I. Summer, Warren R.   II. Title.
    [DNLM: 1. Radiography, Thoracic—Examination Questions.
WF 18.2 A398c 2001]
RC941 .A43 2001
617.5'407572'076—dc21   00-052713

Contents

Preface ix
Acknowledgments xi

Solitary Pulmonary Nodule
Questions 1
Discussions, Answers, and Explanations 10

Multiple Pulmonary Nodules
Questions 15
Discussions, Answers, and Explanations 24

Lung Masses
Questions 27
Discussions, Answers, and Explanations 34

Cavitary Lesions
Questions 37
Discussions, Answers, and Explanations 52

Hyperlucent Lung
Questions 57
Discussions, Answers, and Explanations 70

Cysts and Cystic-Appearing Lesions
Questions 73
Discussions, Answers, and Explanations 82

Diffuse Interstitial Disease
Questions 87
Discussions, Answers, and Explanations 99

DIFFUSE AIRSPACE DISEASE
Questions 105
Discussions, Answers, and Explanations 112

FOCAL AIRSPACE HOMOGENEOUS OPACITIES
Questions 115
Discussions, Answers, and Explanations 124

FOCAL AIRSPACE NONHOMOGENEOUS OPACITIES
Questions 129
Discussions, Answers, and Explanations 140

UNILATERAL COMPLETE OPACIFICATION
Questions 145
Discussions, Answers, and Explanations 150

PLEURAL DISEASE
Questions 153
Discussions, Answers, and Explanations 168

PULMONARY VASCULAR DISEASE
Questions 173
Discussions, Answers, and Explanations 186

MEDIASTINAL COMPARTMENTS
Questions 191
Discussions, Answers, and Explanations 214

CARDIAC AND PERICARDIAL DISEASE
Questions 219
Discussions, Answers, and Explanations 236

CHEST WALL AND SKELETAL DEFORMITIES
Questions 241
Discussions, Answers, and Explanations 254

DIAPHRAGMATIC LESIONS
Questions 257
Discussions, Answers, and Explanations 266

LINES/DEVICES/COMPLICATIONS IN ICU
Questions 269
Discussions, Answers, and Explanations 278

PEDIATRIC CASES
Questions 281
Discussions, Answers, and Explanations 288

LUNG TRANSPLANT PATIENTS
Questions 291
Discussions, Answers, and Explanations 298

Glossary 301

Abbreviations 305

Quick Reference 307

Suggested Reading 311

PREFACE

Chest Radiography: PreTest® Self-Assessment and Review has been designed for medical students and physicians in training. Its basic format parallels the questions in the various steps of the United States Medical Licensing Examinations (USMLE). The design of the book is unique in this series and will serve as a guide for physicians in training. The cases have been compiled on the basis of radiographic patterns and clinical scenarios to enable quicker reference. The Quick Reference guide at the end of the book will help the reader to focus on a particular type of radiographic abnormality and correlate it with a likely applicable clinical scenario. At the same time, this book does not compromise on the basic concept of the PreTest® series and enables the student/reader to prepare for the examination questions that pertain to pulmonary problems within chest x-rays. The clinical items are followed by questions that are based on knowledge of physical examination, associated medical conditions, and broad diagnostic and management strategies to provide a comprehensive educational review. The answers are divided into parts dealing with basic chest radiograph interpretation, followed by a general discussion of related radiographic patterns focused on in that chapter and concluding with the point-by-point answers to specific questions in that chapter. A glossary of terms commonly used in chest radiograph interpretation is also provided to help the reader understand descriptive terms. Thus, this book serves to provide a broadened scope of internal medicine review as well as a medium of instructional learning on how to interpret chest radiographs. It invites the reader to think through the diagnostic and management steps of each case while answering the various components of the questions. This format will also be useful to physicians in training who want to refresh their chest x-ray interpretation techniques in a day-to day clinical setting.

JUZAR ALI, M.D., FRCP(C)

WARREN R. SUMMER, M.D.

Acknowledgments

The authors wish to acknowledge the faculty members of the section of Pulmonary and Critical Care, Department of Medicine, and the Department of Radiology, Louisiana State University Health Sciences Center, for their assistance in compiling the cases and chest radiographs presented in this manuscript.

We dedicate this text to the patients seen at the Medical Center of Louisiana, Charity and University Campus, New Orleans.

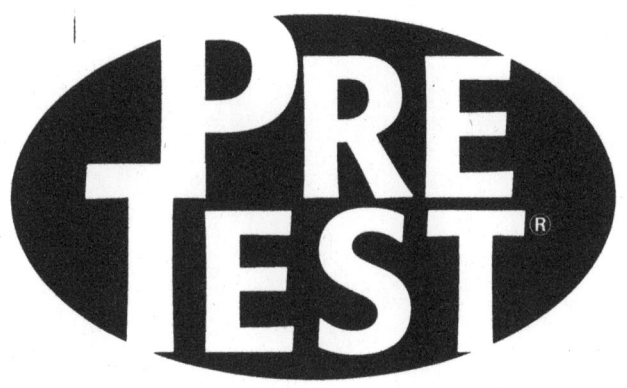

Chest Radiology
PreTest® Self-Assessment and Review

Solitary Pulmonary Nodule

Chest Radiology

DIRECTIONS: Each item below contains a question or incomplete statement followed by suggested responses. Select the **one best** response to each question.

1. A 40-year-old male smoker presents with a history of chronic cough. He has had symptoms of an upper respiratory illness for a few months since visiting family in Arizona. Physical exam is normal. CXR is shown below in Fig. 1. The next step in management should be
    a. Complete pulmonary function tests
    b. Fiberoptic bronchoscopy
    c. Percutaneous needle biopsy
    d. Observation and repeat CXR in 6 to 8 mo

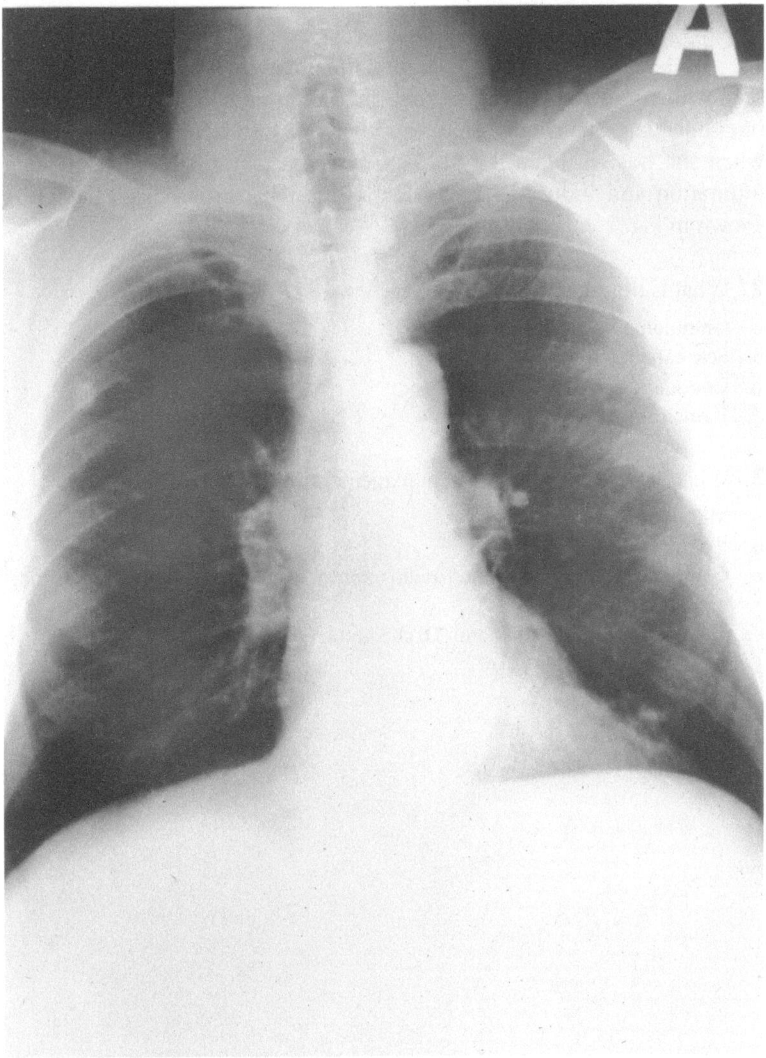

Fig. 1

Items 2–3

A 34-year-old woman, a recent immigrant from Eastern Europe, is seen with complaints of vague chest discomfort after an upper respiratory tract infection. She is not a smoker and gives a history of BCG vaccination when she was an infant. Physical examination is normal. PPD is 10-mm induration and induced sputum for acid-fast bacilli is negative. CXR is shown in Fig. 2.

2. What is the most likely diagnosis?
a. Granuloma
b. Scar carcinoma
c. Coccidioidomycosis
d. Hamartoma

3. What is the next step in the management of this patient?
a. MRI of the chest
b. Fiberoptic bronchoscopy
c. Comparison of previous chest radiograph, if available, and repeat chest radiograph in 3 mo
d. Treatment with four-drug anti-TB chemotherapy

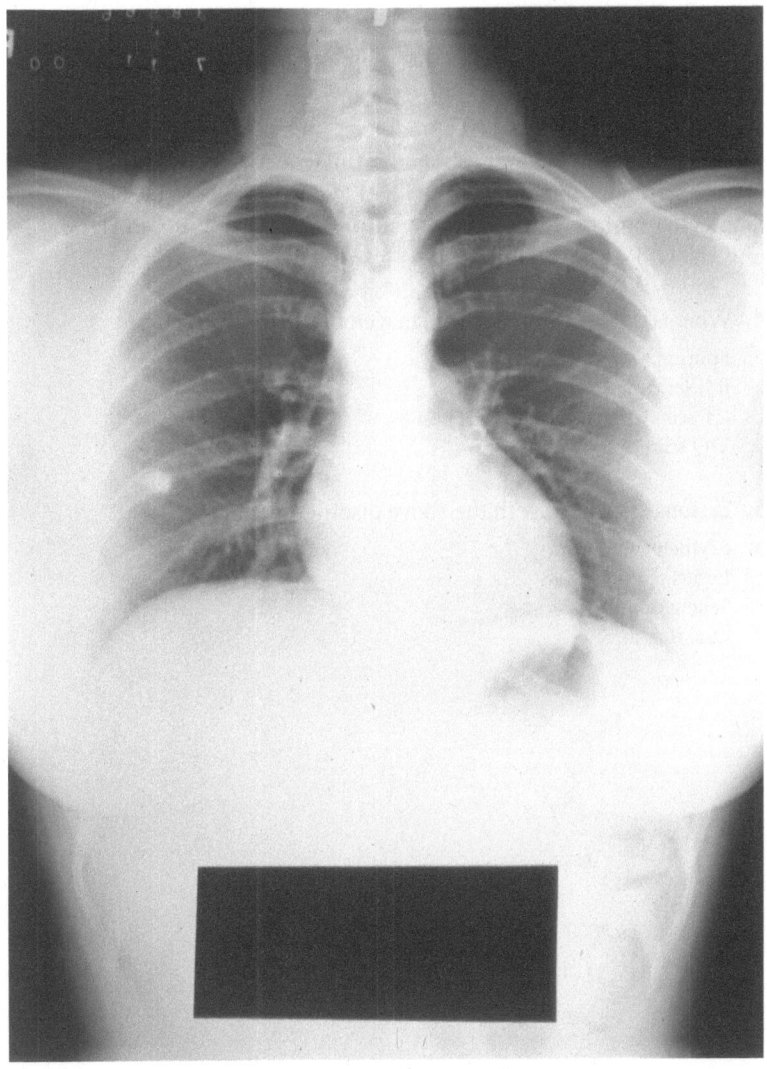

Fig. 2

Items 4–5

A 30-year-old female nonsmoker who recently moved to the U.S. from Mexico presents with dyspnea on exertion. Her PPD is 8 mm. On physical examination, her pulse is 110 bpm, blood pressure is 110/70 mm Hg, and she has mild clubbing, cyanosis, and orthodeoxia. Otherwise, her physical exam is normal. Laboratory data: Hb 14 g/dL; Hct 42%; WBCs 11,000/µL; differential normal. ABGs on room air: pH 7.42; P_{CO_2} 38 mm Hg; P_{O_2} 70 mm Hg. CXR is shown in Fig. 3.

4. What is the next step in the management of this patient?
a. Sputum for fungal culture
b. Rib series
c. CT scan with contrast of the chest
d. V/Q scan

5. Lesions associated with the above disorder include
a. Erythema nodosum
b. Lupus pernio
c. Telangiectasia
d. Oral thrush

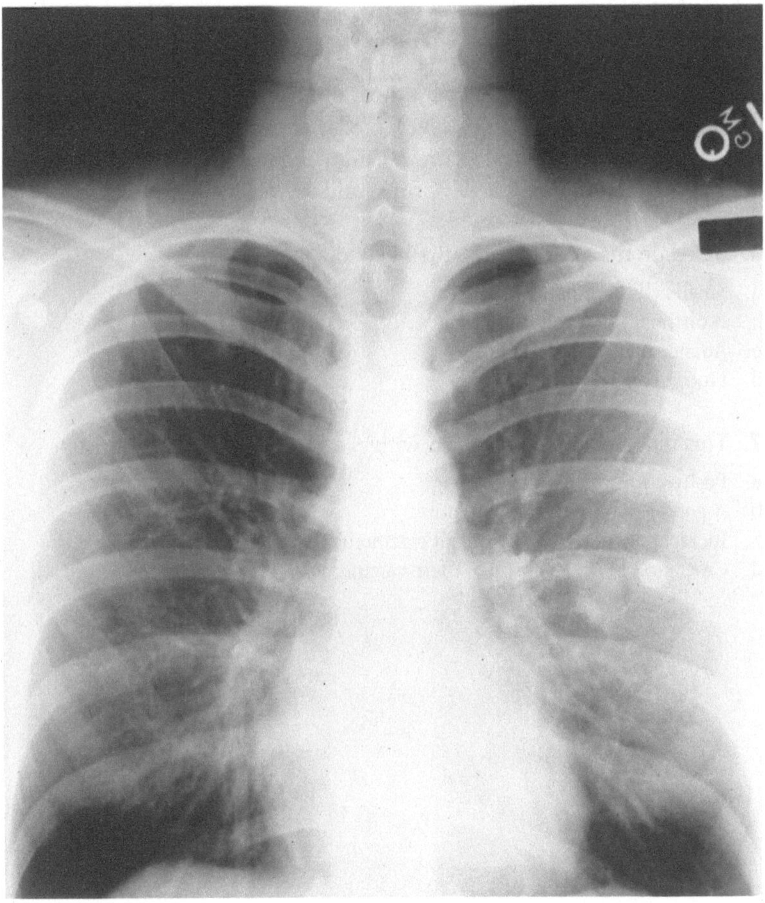

Fig. 3

Items 6–7

A 62-year-old woman with a 30-pack-year smoking history is evaluated with a history of chronic shortness of breath. She has mild left-sided chest discomfort. She denies fever, chills, and night sweats and has no localizing signs on physical exam. A CT-guided needle biopsy of the lesion seen in the CXR in Fig. 4 is performed and reveals malignant cells.

6. Based on the CXR finding, the likely diagnosis is
a. Small cell carcinoma
b. Bronchoalveolar cell carcinoma
c. Adenocarcinoma of the lung
d. Liposarcoma of the chest wall

7. This malignancy is associated with
a. Positive sputum cytology
b. A good response to chemotherapy
c. Incidentally detected peripheral carcinomas on CXR
d. Cavitation in the majority of these carcinomas

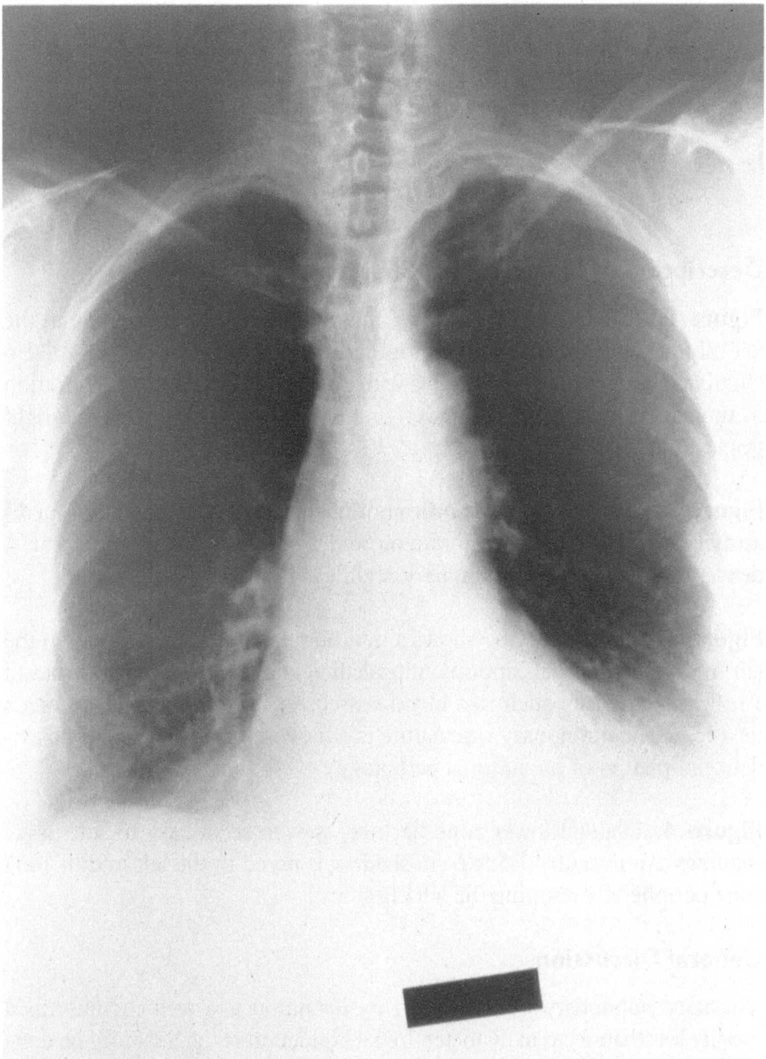

Fig. 4

SOLITARY PULMONARY NODULE

Answers

Description of X-rays in This Chapter

Figure 1. This chest x-ray shows a radiographically dense nodule in the left hilum. Cardiophrenic and costophrenic angles are clear. An 0.8 × 1-cm circular solitary pulmonary nodule with peripheral yet distinct calcification in the superior aspect is seen overlying the 5th posterior rib in the right upper lung zone.

Figure 2. This chest x-ray shows a normal heart size. No pleural or mediastinal disease is noted. Cardiophrenic and costophrenic angles are clear. A dense, rounded solitary pulmonary nodule is noted in the right lung.

Figure 3. This chest x-ray shows a multilobulated nodular opacity in the left midlung zone. This appears noncalcified and has the characteristics of a soft tissue density such as a blood vessel. An ECG monitor lead is seen next to it. The pulmonary vasculature is otherwise normal. There is no evidence of pleural or mediastinal pathology.

Figure 4. Bilateral lower zone haziness is seen secondary to soft tissue shadows. An irregular 1.5 × 2-cm shadow is noted in the left middle lung zone peripherally abutting the left chest wall.

General Discussion

A solitary pulmonary nodule (SPN) by definition is a well-circumscribed opacity less than 3 cm in diameter. Initial evaluation of the SPN may be done in a stepwise fashion. Is this truly an intrapulmonary nodule? Bony shadows such as those originating from the ribs, or soft tissue shadows such as of the nipples, may mimic an SPN. Is this SPN truly solitary? If this is not clear from the chest radiograph or patient examination, a CT scan can be helpful. Comparison with a previous CXR helps avoid unnecessary further workup, as a stable lesion seen on a previous x-ray taken 2 years ago virtually confirms benignity. Small nodules 10 mm or less in size are usually not seen prospectively and may be difficult to find retrospectively on a CXR. Approximately 33% of all SPNs are not detected on an initial radiograph. Evaluation of rate of growth to assess stability of a lesion is helpful to determine benignity. Estimation of doubling time (a 25% increase in diameter is equivalent to doubling of volume) aids in diagnosis. Most bronchogenic carcinomas double within 2 years. Once the diagnosis of SPN has been established, the nodule's characteristics should be evaluated. Characteristics within the nodule such as air bronchograms or cavitation are nonspecific diagnostically. Sharply marginated SPNs are detected more easily. In general, spiculated or ill-defined nodules have a higher incidence of malignancy compared to rounded, smooth-edged nodules. Multilobulated nodules are frequently seen in malignant lesions. Calcification of an SPN is a very helpful feature in differentiating between malignant and benign nodules. The presence of a central or complete calcification virtually excludes malignancy, although eccentric or peripheral calcification may be seen in scar carcinomas. The most common cause of calcified SPNs is old healed granulomatous disease such as TB or fungal disease. Diffuse, stippled "popcorn" calcifications are seen in hamartomas. These are benign mesenchymal lesions of connective tissue origin with mixed fibromuscular/cartilaginous and adipose tissue and are usually discovered as incidental findings in asymptomatic patients. These lesions can grow slowly. Diagnosis is confirmed by thoracotomy. Further evaluation of SPNs depends on patient-related factors such as age and risk factors for cancer. Most cancer is detected after age 55 and is rare before age 35. Diagnostic tests such as CT-guided transthoracic biopsy or fiberoptic bronchoscopy are done based on the accessibility of the lesion by these approaches. Central lesions with air bronchograms leading to them are more accessible by bronchoscopy, whereas a CT-guided needle aspiration/biopsy has a better yield in peripheral lesions. Surgical therapeutic options in SPNs that are determined to be malignant or nondiagnostic by noninvasive procedures in patients at high risk for cancer depend upon mediastinal involvement and staging. Preoperative staging of lung tumors is done either by CT scan and/or mediastinoscopy.

Specific Discussion

1. The answer is c. Based on the age of the patient, risk factors, and persistent symptoms, further diagnostic tests are warranted. Observation for 6 mo is inappropriate. Due to the peripheral nature of this lesion, a CT-guided needle biopsy would be the best diagnostic strategy and have a better yield than a bronchoscopy. Pulmonary function tests would be helpful if surgery is planned, but would not alter the diagnostic steps. In this case, the CT-guided biopsy revealed coccidioidomycosis. This is caused by a fungus (*Coccidioides immitis*) in the soil and is seen in desert semiarid climates with a short, intense rainy season. It is endemic in southwestern North America, Mexico, and Central and South America. Most patients are asymptomatic or recover fully after initial flulike illness. The radiographic findings of coccidioidomycosis are variable and depend upon the severity of the disease. Most granulomas are smaller than 2 cm, and almost all are less than 3 cm in size. Besides SPNs, in the early stages of coccidioidomycosis patchy infiltrates may be accompanied by hilar and mediastinal adenopathy and less frequently by pleural effusion. In cases of persistent disease, infiltrates may enlarge.

2–3. The answers are 2-a, 3-c. With a history of a positive PPD in a young immigrant and the presence of a calcified peripheral SPN, the likely diagnosis is tuberculous granuloma. Comparison with a previous x-ray to confirm stability of the lesion would prevent the need for further diagnostic tests. An MRI of the chest would not add definitive information, and bronchoscopy for a peripherally located calcified lesion would be of low yield. Since this lesion probably represents latent, old, healed granulomatous focus, treatment with four antituberculosis drugs is not warranted unless evidence of active disease is seen.

4–5. The answers are 4-c, 5-c. The clinical picture with orthodeoxia (oxygen desaturation in an erect position) suggests an arteriovenous malformation (AVM). Congenital pulmonary AVMs of the lung represent a direct communication between the pulmonary arteries and the veins, bypassing the capillary bed and resulting in cyanosis due to right-to-left shunt. Dyspnea and hemoptysis are common clinical presentations. Fifty percent of AVMs are associated with Osler-Weber-Rendu syndrome (AVMs with mucosal telangiectasias). The chest x-ray shows a multilobulated opacity and the feeding vessels are characteristically seen on a CT scan. The definitive diagnostic test is an angiogram.

6–7. The answers are 6-c, 7-c. An SPN in a 42-year-old smoker mandates a diagnostic workup. In this case, a CT-guided biopsy revealed malignant cells. Adenocarcinoma is commonly peripheral and represents about 30% of the total number of lung cancer cases. Its incidence is rising especially in females. Adenocarcinoma frequently presents as an incidental finding on x-ray. The other major histological types of lung cancer tend to have central localization and are as follows:

1. Squamous (epidermoid) carcinoma. Eighty percent are central; when peripheral, they have a tendency for cavitation.
2. Small cell (oat cell) carcinoma. Believed to originate from neuroendocrine cells of the bronchial mucosa, these are usually central with mediastinal involvement.
3. Large cell undifferentiated carcinoma with mixed malignant features.
4. Bronchoalveolar carcinoma. A variant of adenocarcinoma, these arise from type II pneumocytes in the alveoli. They may simulate pneumonia with focal consolidation or may present as solitary or multiple nodules.

Multiple Pulmonary Nodules

Chest Radiology

DIRECTIONS: Each item below contains a question or incomplete statement followed by suggested responses. Select the **one best** response to each question.

Items 8–9

A 71-year-old man is seen with low-grade fever, generalized malaise, and a run-down feeling. He has lost weight and shows stigmata of chronic illness. There is no history of occupational exposure. On physical examination, vital signs are as follows: pulse 110 bpm; temperature 99°F; respirations 19/min; blood pressure 90/60 mm Hg. On exam, the man is frail and appears cachectic with temporal wasting. Other aspects of his physical exam are unremarkable. Laboratory data: Hb 10 g/dL; Hct 30%; MCV 90; WBCs 3000/μL; differential normal; BUN 19 mg/dL; creatinine 1.0 mg/dL; sodium 129 mEq/L; potassium 5.0 mEq/L; ABGs (RA): pH 7.42, P_{CO_2} 35 mm Hg, P_{O_2} 58 mm Hg. Spirometry: FVC 60% of predicted; FEV_1 60% of predicted. PPD skin test is negative (0 mm); induced sputum for AFB smear is negative. Chest radiograph is shown below in Fig. 5.

8. What is the most likely diagnosis?

a. Silicosis
b. Miliary TB
c. Metastatic thyroid carcinoma
d. Sarcoidosis

9. What is the next step in the workup of this patient that would most likely yield the diagnosis?

a. CT scan of the chest
b. Thyroid function tests
c. Bone marrow aspiration for culture
d. Thoracoscopic lung biopsy

Multiple Pulmonary Nodules 17

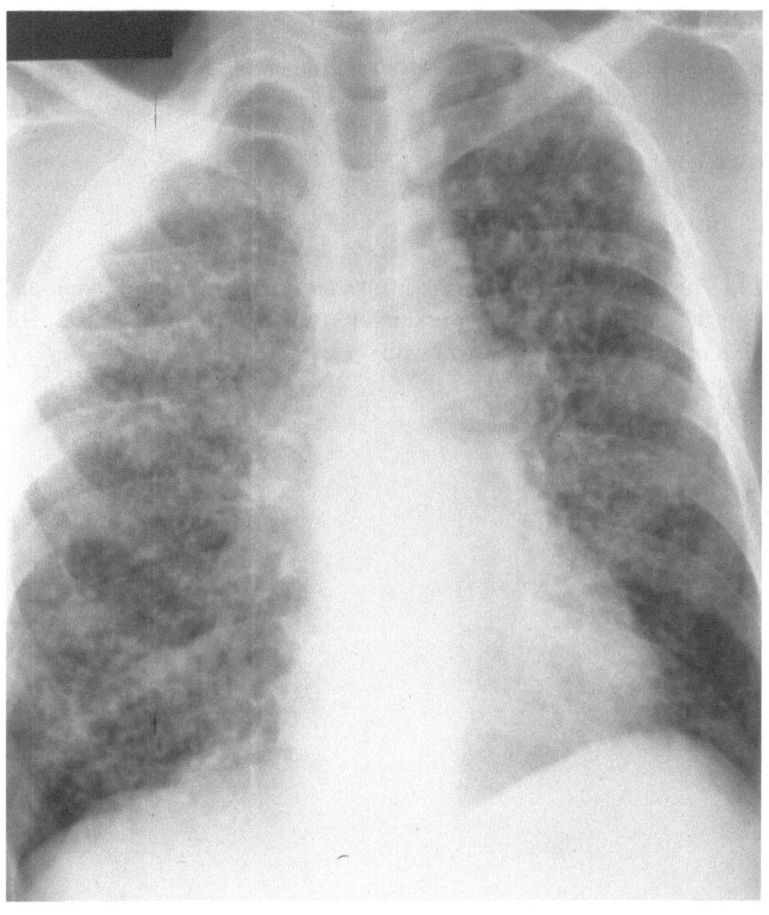

Fig. 5

Items 10–11

10. Based on the CXR shown in Fig. 6, all of the following may be helpful in the diagnosis except
   a. Occupational history
   b. Sputum for AFB
   c. Sputum for fungus
   d. History of rheumatic fever

11. This patient's occupational history reveals exposure to iron ore, asphalt, and dust related to working on loading docks for 10 years. The CXR in Fig. 6 is most consistent with
   a. Silicosis
   b. Asbestosis
   c. Bagassosis
   d. Chlorine gas exposure

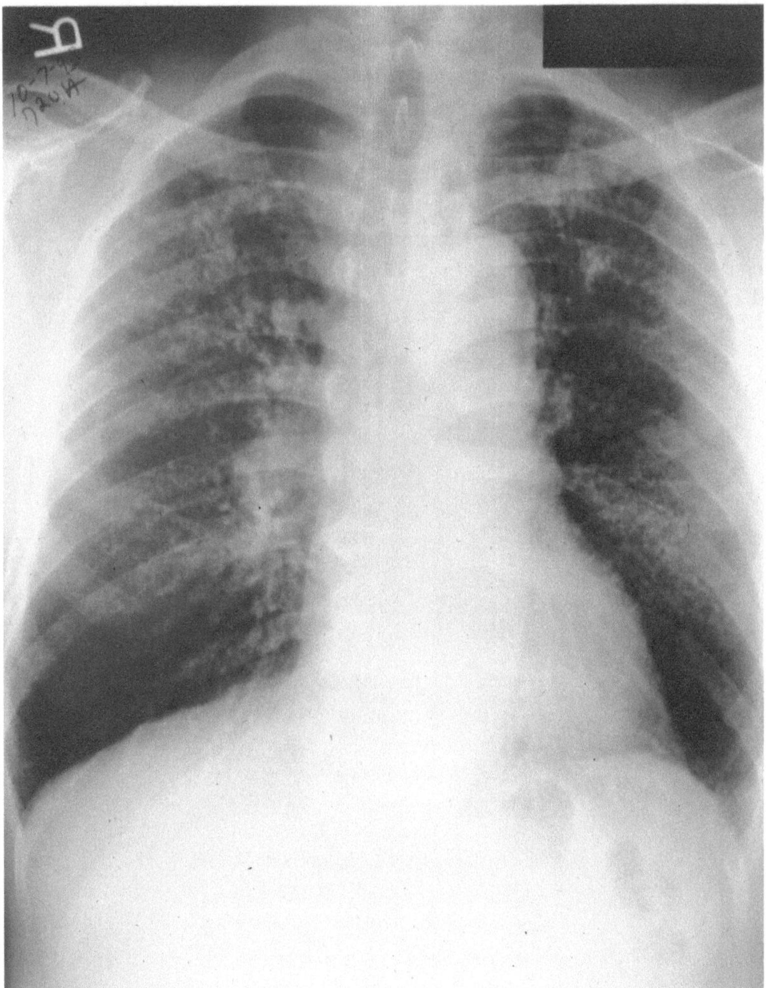

Fig. 6

12. A 70-year-old man with a history of emphysema and progressive dyspnea is admitted with mild hemoptysis. On exam, he is afebrile; he has a left-sided chest wall scar from a previous thoracotomy with decreased breath sounds in the left lung field. There are wheezes and rhonchi heard in the right lung field. The CXR is shown in Fig. 7. Based on the CXR and clinical history, the most likely diagnosis is

a. Left lung atelectasis with mucus plug
b. Metastatic lung disease from lung primary
c. Multiple pulmonary infarcts
d. Septic emboli

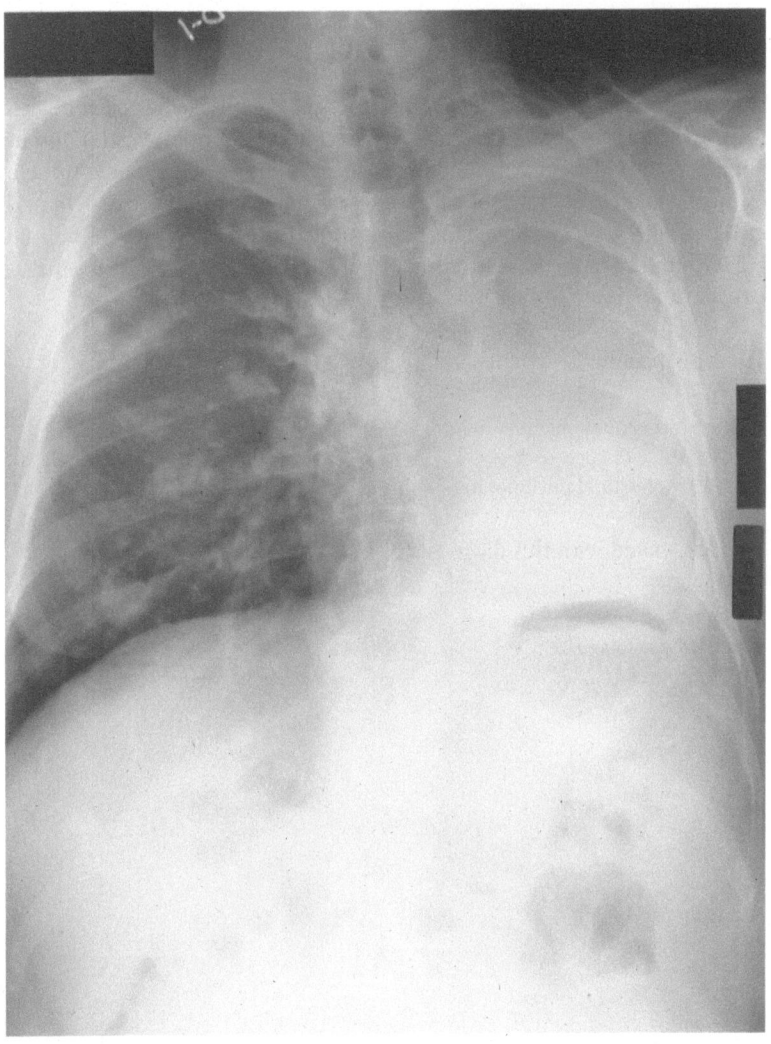

Fig. 7

Items 13-14

A 53-year-old male smoker, unemployed with no occupational exposure, is admitted with progressive shortness of breath. He has been unwell for some time and has received multiple courses of antibiotics for "bronchitis." During the prior 4 mo, he has not had any medical follow-up. On exam, he is afebrile but looks ill. Lung exams reveal diffuse rhonchi and crackles with no localizing signs. ABGs on room air show PaO_2 of 68 mm Hg with mild compensated respiratory alkalosis. Sputum for AFB is negative. CXR is shown in Fig. 8.

13. The most likely diagnosis is
a. TB
b. Hypersensitivity pneumonitis
c. Metastatic disease
d. Acute interstitial pneumonitis

14. Associated with this diagnosis is
a. Clubbing
b. Increased IgE
c. Hypocalcemia
d. Eosinophilia

Multiple Pulmonary Nodules

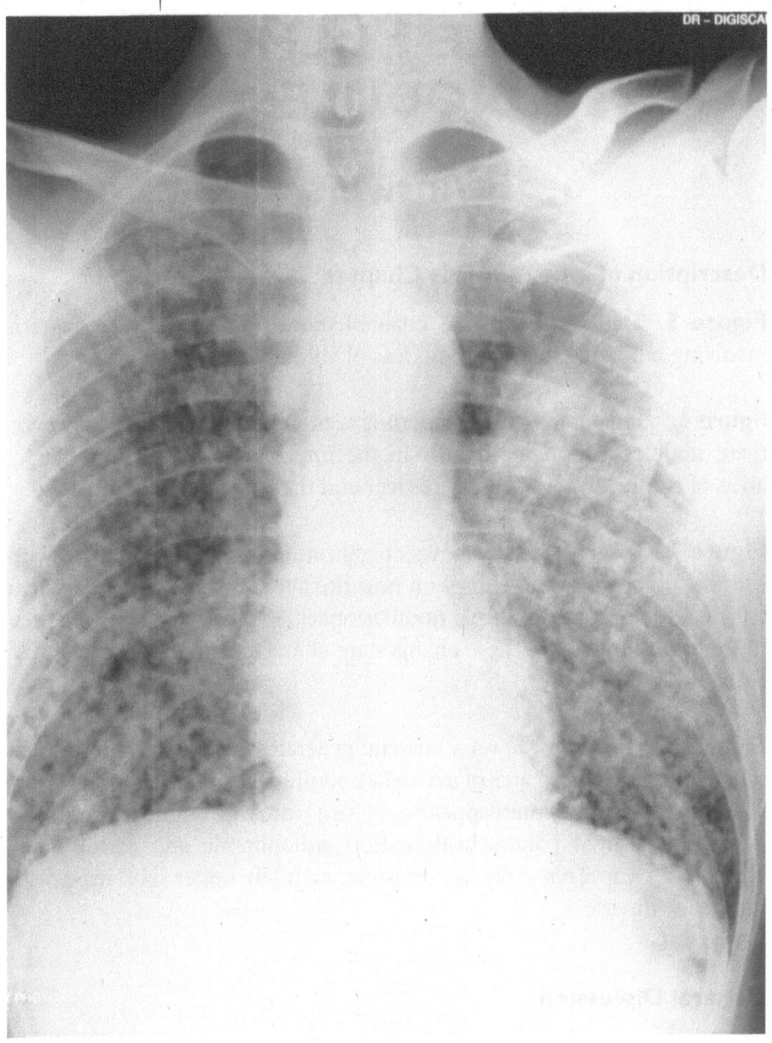

Fig. 8

MULTIPLE PULMONARY NODULES

Answers

Description of X-rays in This Chapter

Figure 5. This x-ray shows a bilateral diffuse miliary nodular pattern involving both lung fields with no loss of volume.

figure 6. A bilateral nodular pattern is seen in both lung fields. However, these nodules are predominantly in the upper zones with some patchy areas of confluence. The bases are clear and there is no pleural disease.

Figure 7. This chest x-ray shows opacification of the left lung field with surgical rib changes and clips seen near the left main stem secondary to a left pneumonectomy. Multiple nodular opacities of varying sizes are seen in the right lung field. These changes are characteristic of metastatic disease.

Figure 8. This x-ray shows a bilateral generalized nodular pattern in all lung fields. There is an area of a masslike confluence in the left upper zone. The superior mediastinum appears widened primarily on the left side with a prominent right paratracheal node. Cardiophrenic and costophrenic angles are clear. This x-ray is consistent with left upper lobe mass with metastatic disease.

General Discussion

Characteristically, miliary nodules are less than 4 mm in size. They are generally noncalcified and diffuse and are seen in many conditions, such as TB/fungal infections/pneumoconiosis and certain malignancies such as melanomas/thyroid cancer. Larger, more confluent lesions can be seen in alveolar sarcoid, Wegener's granulomatosis, and metastatic disease. The clinical hints that aid diagnosis include:

- An occupational history without constitutional symptoms.
- X-ray that looks worse than the patient's complaints, as in sarcoidosis.
- History of thromboembolic disease or sepsis, as in septic emboli or pulmonary infarcts. These are generally seen in the lower lung zones.
- History of arthritis; may suggest rheumatoid nodules.
- Presence of eosinophilia in the peripheral smear with fleeting infiltrates; provides clue for pulmonary infiltrates with eosinophilia (PIE) syndrome, in which case history of travel or use of medications/drugs may be helpful and a stool exam may aid in the diagnosis.
- Immune-compromised patients may have opportunistic infections such as herpes or CMV.

Specific Discussion

8–9. The answers are 8-b, 9-d. This elderly patient has all the stigmata of chronic illness. Although the PPD skin test and sputum studies are negative (seen in about 30% of cases), the history and CXR are consistent with miliary TB. Hyponatremia and hypercalcemia are common findings in TB. In this age group sarcoidosis is unlikely. In the absence of occupational exposure, silicosis is also unlikely. Bone marrow aspirate may be positive for TB culture in 60% of patients with miliary TB, and aspiration is a logical step in the diagnostic evaluation. CT scan will not aid further in the diagnosis, and thyroid function tests will be normal unless there is clinical evidence of hypo- or hyperthyroidism. Open lung or thoracoscopic biopsy is always diagnostic.

10–11. The answers are 10-d, 11-a. The CXR differential warrants consideration of all the diagnostic choices outlined except rheumatic fever. Silicosis is caused by inhalation of silica dioxide dust. Exposed populations include sandblasters, stone grinders, ceramic workers, and mine workers. Acute silicosis, also called silicoproteinosis, can rarely develop after a single massive exposure and results in pulmonary consolidation. Simple silicosis causes multiple discrete pulmonary nodules occurring with upper zone predominance. Mediastinal adenopathy is common and classically seen with "eggshell" calcification. Complicated silicosis or progressive massive fibrosis refers to larger confluent densities or conglomerate upper lobe masses. Patients usually have progressive functional impairment, and cor pulmonale is common. Tuberculosis occurs with increased incidence in silicosis, and a positive PPD in such patients with no evidence of active disease warrants chemoprophylaxis. Bagassosis due to exposure to sugar cane residue presents with a hypersensitivity pneumonitis, and chlorine gas exposure causes upper airway dysfunction. Pulmonary chlorine gas injury requires exposure in a confined space and is followed by pulmonary leak syndrome (ARDS) and bronchiolitis. Asbestosis refers to respiratory dysfunction and impairment and pathologic changes seen in the lung parenchyma characterized by increased interstitial changes in the lower zones. Other radiographic evidence of asbestos exposure includes pleural plaques and pleural and pericardial calcification.

12. The answer is b. With the history of a left-sided thoracotomy and chest radiograph changes consistent with a pneumonectomy, the right-sided lesions are most likely metastatic lung cancer. There is no clinical evidence of a mucus plug with atelectasis, although the roentgenographic picture of a homogeneous density without air bronchogram with an ipsilateral mediastinal shift is typical of lung atelectasis. The history does not support other choices.

13–14. The answers are 13-c, 14-a. This clinical scenario is consistent with metastatic carcinoma. The presence of a confluent density in the left upper lobe suggests the metastases probably arose from a lung primary malignancy. Diffuse pulmonary nodular metastases usually arise from a nonlung primary (70%). Clubbing is the most likely associated finding. Hypocalcemia is unlikely. Hypercalcemia is most commonly caused by bony metastases, especially with small cell carcinoma and adenocarcinoma. It is seen in squamous cell carcinoma as a result of humoral mediators with PTH-like activity. However, squamous cell carcinoma of the lung is a very infrequent cause of widespread pulmonary metastasis. Sputum for AFB would most likely be positive in this radiographic setting. Eosinophilia and increased IgE levels may be seen in the pulmonary infiltrates with eosinophilia syndrome, but there is no indication or history of fleeting infiltrates to support that diagnosis here.

Lung Masses

Chest Radiology

DIRECTIONS: Each item below contains a question or incomplete statement followed by suggested responses. Select the **one best** response to each question.

15. A 60-year-old man with a past history of smoking for 30 years (he stopped 3 years ago, prior to cardiac bypass surgery) is admitted with cough and mild hemoptysis. He is afebrile with no shortness on breath. Physical exam is negative except that the lung exam reveals rhonchi in the left upper lung zone. The finding/abnormality most likely to occur with the lesion seen on the CXR in Fig. 9 is
   a. Serum calcium of 13.6 mg/dL
   b. Sputum positive for fungal elements
   c. Increased D-dimer levels
   d. Koilonychia

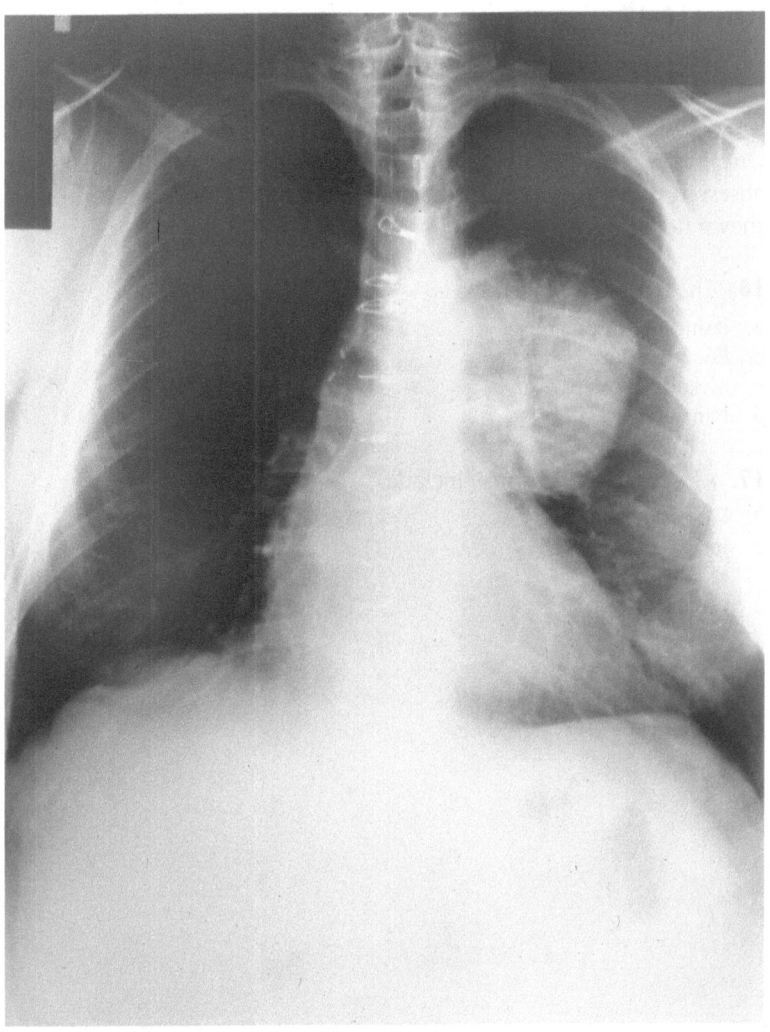

Fig. 9

Items 16–17

A 38-year-old city worker presents with fever, chills, and cough with left-sided chest pain 2 days after the Mardi Gras festival. She denies any hemoptysis, weight loss, or chronic illness. Past history is unremarkable. On physical exam, she has a BMI of 32; temperature is 101°F. She was observed to have splinting of her right side during the inspiration CXR shown in Fig. 10.

16. The most likely diagnosis is

a. Bronchogenic carcinoma
b. Round pneumonia
c. Alveolar sarcoidosis
d. Fungus ball

17. Associated findings may include

a. Hyponatremia
b. Increased ACE levels
c. Hypercalcemia
d. Clubbing

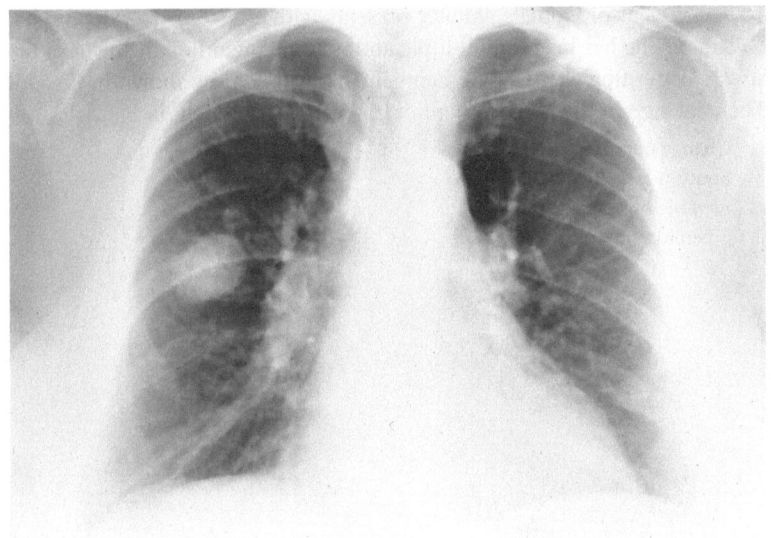

Fig. 10

18. A 62-year-old female smoker presents with a history of "pneumonia" 6 wk ago. She has been on multiple antibiotics, and although she feels relatively better now, her CXR remains unchanged. CXR is shown in Fig. 11. The next step in the management of this patient will include

a. Change of antibiotics
b. Sputum for TB
c. Flexible bronchoscopy
d. Open lung biopsy

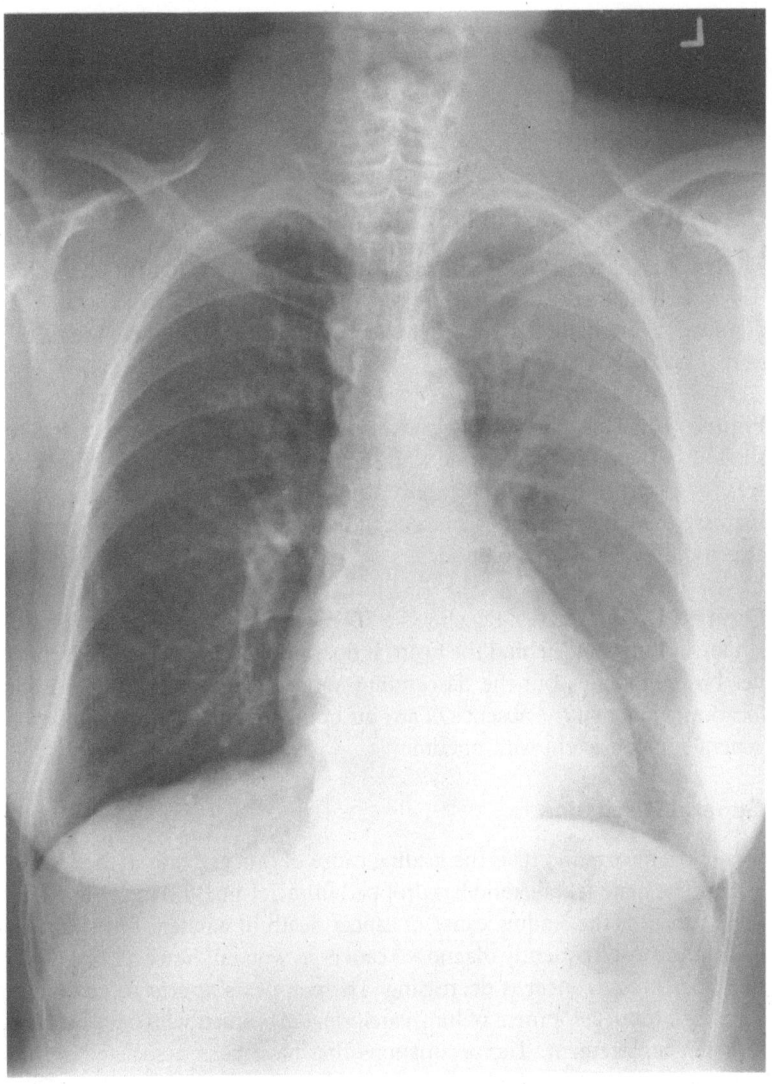

Fig. 11

Lung Masses

Answers

Description of X-rays in This Chapter

Figure 9. A large, 7 × 11-cm mass is seen in the left parahilar area. This has a well-defined edge and silhouettes out the hilar structures. The diaphragms are flattened, and there is no pleural disease. There are mediastinal (sternal) wires from prior CABG.

Figure 10. This chest x-ray shows a 3 × 2.5-cm rounded masslike shadow in the right middle zone with slightly irregular margins. There is an area of nonspecific infiltrate above this mass with air bronchograms. Increased vascular markings are seen in the right lower zone and the hilar area reveals calcified lymph nodes.

Figure 11. This chest x-ray shows a 7 × 4-cm oval-shaped opacity in the left lower lung zone behind the heart. It does not obscure the left heart border but silhouettes out the descending aorta, documenting its posterior location. Note that the absence of any air bronchograms within the mass is generally inconsistent with pneumonia.

General Discussion

Bronchogenic carcinoma is the leading cause of cancer death in the United States. The male-female ratio has dropped from 7:1 in 1960 to 2:1 in 1998. Lung cancer is the leading cause of cancer death in women. Breast cancer is still the most frequently diagnosed cancer in women; however, the death rate from breast cancer is decreasing. There appears appear to be an elevated risk for development of lung carcinoma in women who have been on estrogen replacement. The occupations that have been associated with a high rate of lung cancer include nurse, cashier, waitress, and orderly. Data suggests that excess smoking prevalence in these occupations is part of the risk. Women are more susceptible to the carcinogens in tobacco smoke than men; this may be due in part to lower plasma clearance of nicotine in women. Also, the P450 system is more active in men and therefore the breakdown in oxidative capacity is more active in men. Women develop more DNA damage at lower smoker exposure levels. Twenty-five percent of lung cancer patients have no symptoms at the time of diagnosis. Usual symptoms include cough, shortness of breath, hemoptysis, wheezing, and paraneoplastic syndromes that may bring the patient to medical attention. Ten percent of heavy smokers will develop lung cancer. Cigarette smoking is commonly associated with squamous cell carcinoma, small cell carcinoma, and, to a lesser degree, adenocarcinoma. Other carcinogens include asbestos, heavy metal, radiation, and urban pollutants. Radiographically, a peripheral mass is the most common manifestation of adenocarcinoma. Squamous cell carcinomas attain large size and frequently cavitate, and patients may present with lung collapse and consolidation distal to a central obstruction. Small cell carcinoma typically presents with a proximal mass, lymphadenopathy, and mediastinal invasion.

Specific Discussion

15. The answer is a. This CXR is consistent with a bronchogenic carcinoma and is likely to be associated with hypercalcemia if this is small cell or squamous cell carcinoma. The clinical findings are not consistent with fungal disease or thromboembolism. The chest x-ray in fungal infection is usually multi-segmental, and pulmonary embolism tends to cause patchy infiltrates with pleural effusion. Koilonychia is spoon-shaped nails seen in severe iron-deficiency anemia.

16–17. The answers are 16-b, 17-a. The history is classical for a community-acquired pneumonia. The radiographic pattern seen in pneumonia includes ill-defined opacities with air bronchograms in a segmental or lobar distribution. However, rounded densities can sometimes be seen in both typical and atypical pneumonia. Infections such as pneumonias and TB may be associated with hyponatremia due to inappropriate ADH secretion.

18. The answer is c. The CXR shows a masslike density in the left lower lobe. Change of antibiotics would be inappropriate; TB seldom presents with this radiographic picture. With the history of a nonresolving opacity and protracted treatment with antibiotics being unsuccessful, further diagnostic steps are needed. A CT would help define location and exclude sequestration or a posterior mediastinal mass. As a first step, bronchoscopy and evaluation of the airways would probably yield a histopathologic diagnosis in this endobronchial and intrapulmonary lesion. Open lung biopsy would be indicated only if bronchoscopy and other studies are nondiagnostic.

Cavitary Lesions

Chest Radiology

DIRECTIONS: Each item below contains a question or incomplete statement followed by suggested responses. Select the **one best** response to each question.

Items 19–20

A 40-year-old man with a history of substance abuse and HIV infection is seen in the ER with complaints of fever, weight loss, production of foul-smelling sputum, and shortness of breath for 2 wk. On physical exam he is tachypneic and has clubbing of his digits. Lung exam reveals diffuse rhonchi and an area of egophony with whispering pectoriloquy in the right chest posteriorly. ABGs reveal PaO_2 of 59 mm Hg on room air. CXR is shown in Fig. 12.

19. What is the most likely diagnosis?
a. Pneumococcal pneumonia
b. PCP pneumonia
c. Lung abscess
d. Squamous cell carcinoma

20. What is the next step in management of this patient?
a. Give antibiotics to cover mixed aerobic and anaerobic infection
b. Determine serum LDH level
c. Perform immediate bronchoscopy
d. Give antibiotics to cover community-acquired pneumonia

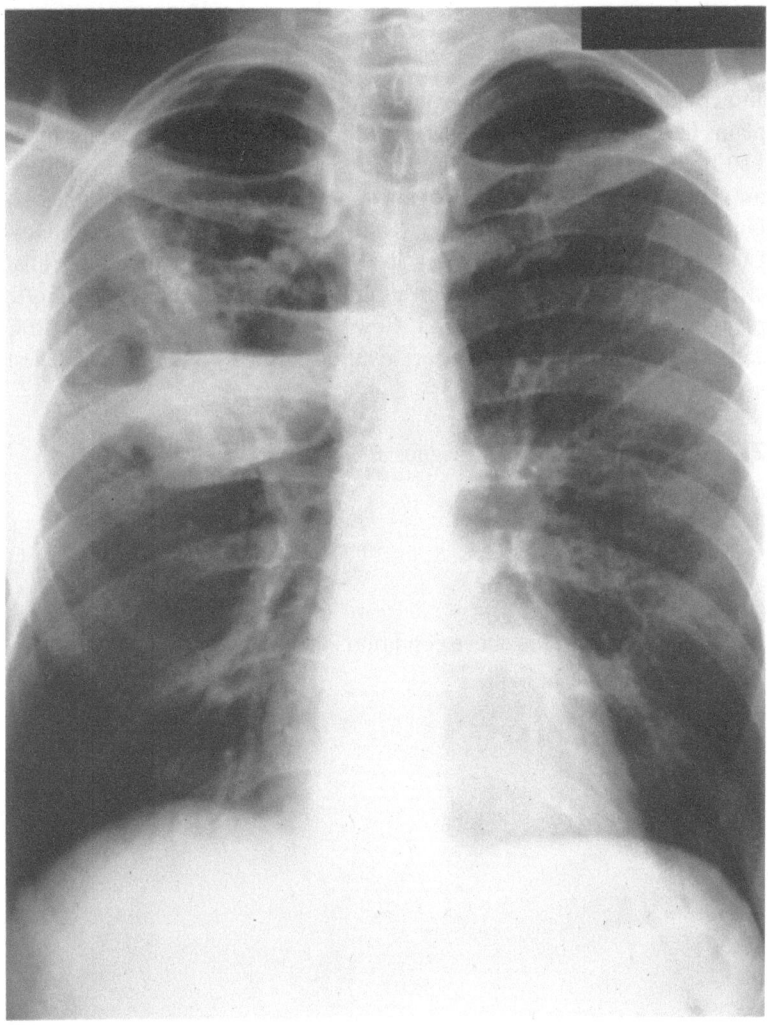

Fig. 12

Items 21–22

A 50-year-old woman is seen with symptoms of progressive dyspnea and cough productive of yellow sputum mixed with blood. She also complains of nasal discharge, arthalgias, and low-grade fever. Vital signs: pulse 110 bpm; temperature 99°F; respirations 19/min; blood pressure 140/90 mm Hg. On general exam, the patient appears ill with crusty nasal mucosa. Lung exam reveals diffuse crackles with nonlocalized areas of egophony. Laboratory data: Hb 12 g/dL; Hct 36%; WBCs 12.8/μL with a differential of 15% bands; BUN 30 mg/dL; creatinine 1.6 mg/dL; sodium 138 mEq/L; potassium 4.2 mEq/L. Urinalysis shows 3+ protein with RBC and RBC casts and negative leukocyte esterase. Sputum for AFB is negative. Chest x-ray is shown below in Fig. 13.

21. What is the most likely diagnosis?
a. Lung abscess
b. Wegener's granulomatosis
c. Squamous cell cancer
d. TB

22. Associated with the above condition is
a. High rheumatoid factor titers
b. Positive C-ANCA
c. Increased ACE levels
d. Clubbing

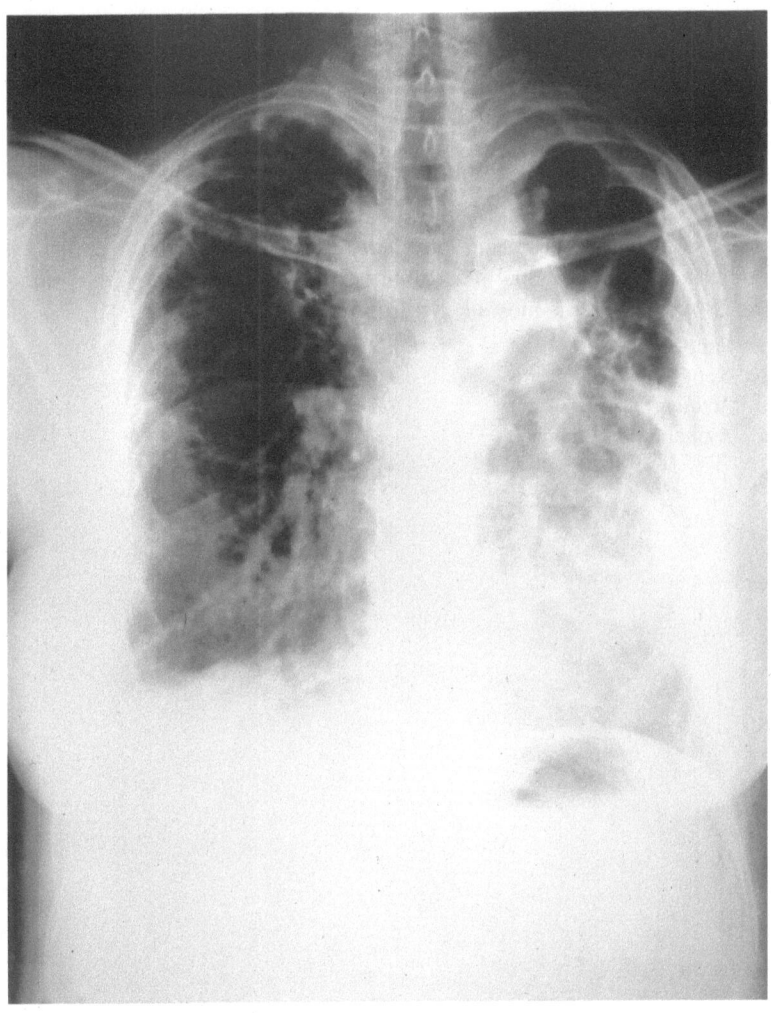

Fig. 13

23. A 60-year-old man with a history of COPD and old TB is seen with mild hemoptysis and chronic cough. He is HIV negative and has been ill for about 2 wk. Vital signs: pulse 110 bpm; temperature 101°F; respirations 24/min; blood pressure 108/70 mm Hg. No skin lesions are noted. Laboratory data: Hb 14 g/dL; HCA 42%; WBCs 8.7/µL; BUN 24 mg/dL; creatinine 0.8 mg/dL; sodium 131 mEq/L; potassium 4.3 mEq/L. ABGs on RA: pH 7.37; P_{CO_2} 43 mm Hg; P_{O_2} 87 mm Hg. Sputum tests reveal numerous AFB-positive organisms on smear. Spirometry shows an obstructive ventilatory impairment with marginal reversibility. CXR is shown in Fig. 14. Among the choices listed, the most likely diagnosis is

a. Lung abscess
b. Non-TB mycobacteria
c. Actinomycosis
d. Aspiration pneumonia

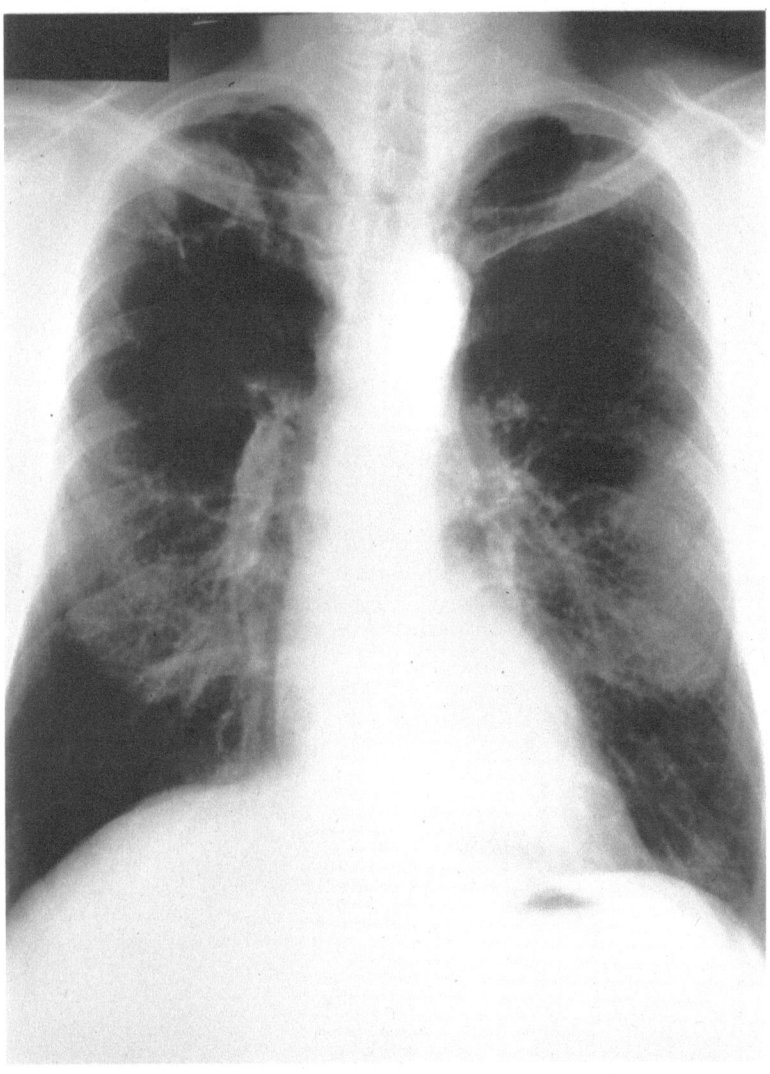

Fig. 14

Notes

Items 24–25

A 49-year-old woman with no smoking history presents with a sudden bout of hemoptysis reported to be about 600 cc, increasing cough, and dyspnea on exertion. She was diagnosed with sarcoidosis in the past and has been on steroid treatment off and on. Her last cycle of steroids was 2 years ago. She complains of episodes of mild intermittent hemoptysis over the last 2 mo not associated with URI symptoms or purulent sputum. On physical examination, vital signs are: pulse 106 bpm; temperature 100°F; respirations 34/min; blood pressure 110/68 mm Hg. On general examination, the patient appears in moderate distress, and pertinent findings include crackles heard in the left upper lung zones. Laboratory data: Hb 11.2 g/dL; Hct 33%; WBCs 10.9/μL with lymphopenia; BUN 34 mg/dL; creatinine 0.9 mg/dL; sodium 126 mEq/L; potassium 5.6 mEq/L; PPD negative. PFTs performed 6 mo ago show: FVC 1.8 (45% of predicted); FEV 1.0.8.L (34% of predicted); DLCO 46% of predicted. CXR is shown in Fig. 15a; CT scan is shown in Fig. 15b.

24. What is the most likely diagnosis?
a. Sarcoidosis exacerbation
b. Cavitary carcinoma
c. Lung abscess
d. Aspergilloma

25. The therapeutic step most likely to result in the control of bleeding is
a. Restarting of steroids
b. IV amphotericin
c. Intracavitary itraconazole
d. Bronchial artery embolization

Chest Radiology

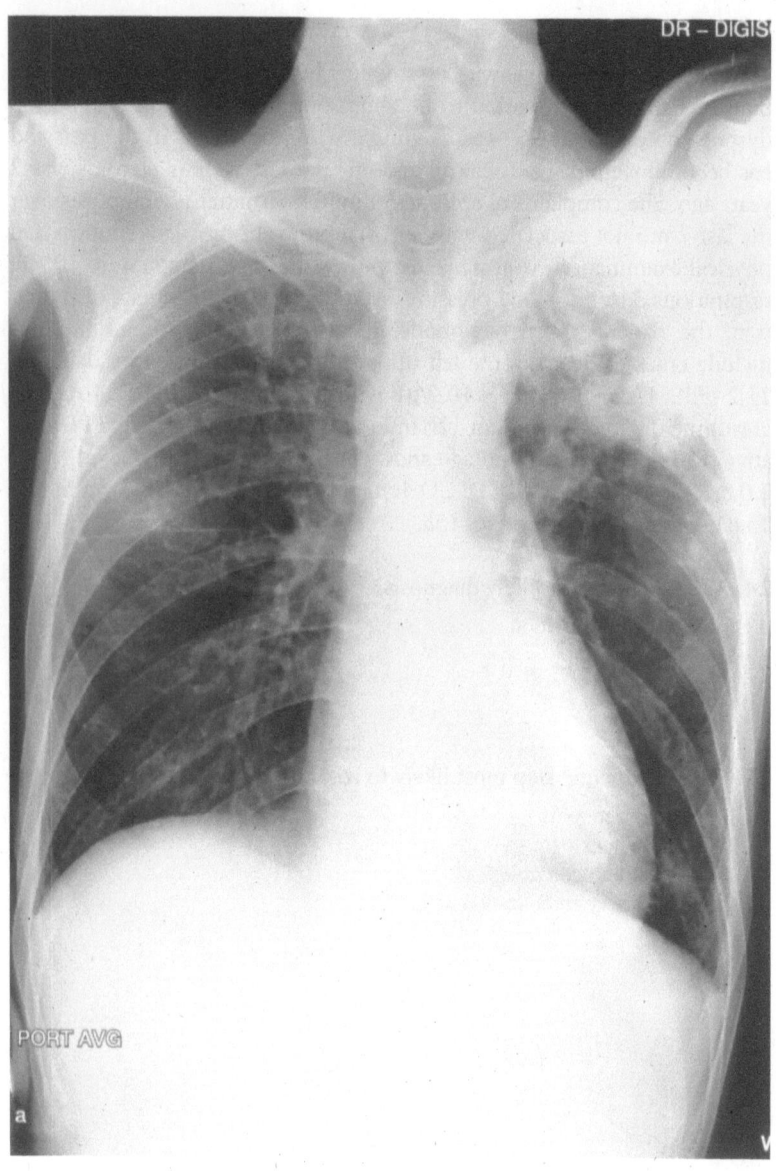

Fig. 15a

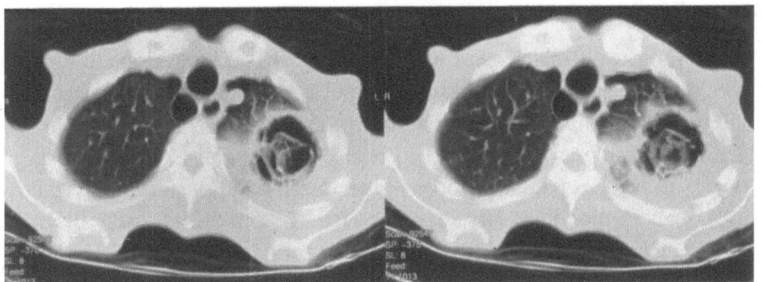

Fig. 15b

Items 26–27

A 42-year-old black man with a history of IVDA develops low-grade fever, night sweats, weight loss, cough, and hemoptysis. On physical examination, vital signs are: pulse 109 bpm; temperature 100°F; respirations 22/min; blood pressure 110/70 mm Hg. On general exam, the patient appears ill and has palpable nodes in the anterior and posterior cervical triangle. Laboratory data: Hb 11 g/dL; Hct 32%; WBCs 7.2/µL; BUN 12 mg/dL; creatinine 0.3 mg/dL; sodium 129 mEq/L; potassium 3.2 mEq/L; LDH 217 IU/L; PPD negative. ABGs on RA: pH 7.4; P_{CO_2} 34 mm Hg; P_{O_2} 66 mm Hg. Chest radiograph is shown below in Fig. 16.

26. What is the most likely diagnosis?
a. TB
b. Lymphoma
c. Sarcoidosis
d. Mycetoma

27. What is the next management option?
a. Obtain ACE level
b. Start four-drug anti-TB treatment
c. Start antifungal treatment
d. Repeat PPD and start INH chemoprophylaxis

Cavitary Lesions 49

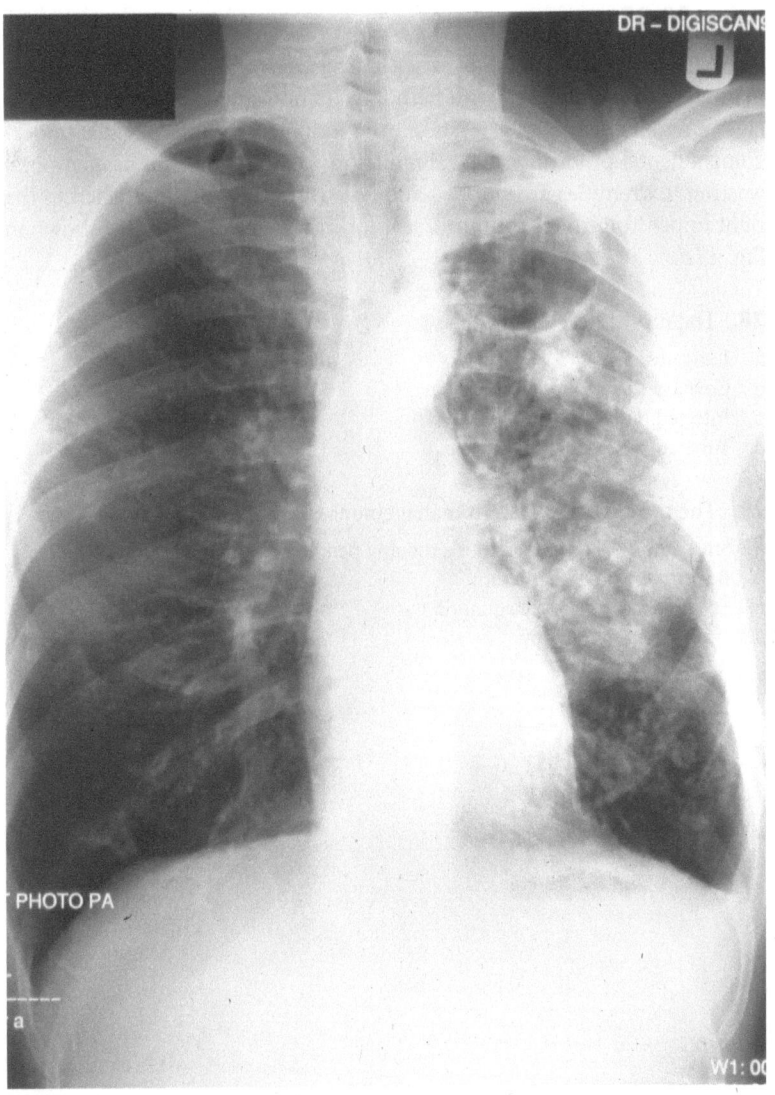

Fig. 16

Items 28–29

A 56-year-old male smoker with a history of chronic dry cough for many months is admitted with hemoptysis and significant weight loss. He gives a remote history of aspiration of a tooth many years ago while undergoing a dental procedure. On examination, he is afebrile and has temporal wasting. Extremities are clubbed and breath sounds are diminished in the right upper lung zone. Sputum smear for AFB is negative. CXR is shown in Fig. 17.

28. The most likely diagnosis is
a. Lung abscess
b. Cavitary squamous cell carcinoma
c. Infected bulla
d. Tuberculosis

29. The next specific step in management is
a. Start empirical antituberculosis therapy pending culture data
b. Begin chest physical therapy
c. Schedule a surgical consultation
d. Perform bronchoscopy

Cavitary Lesions 51

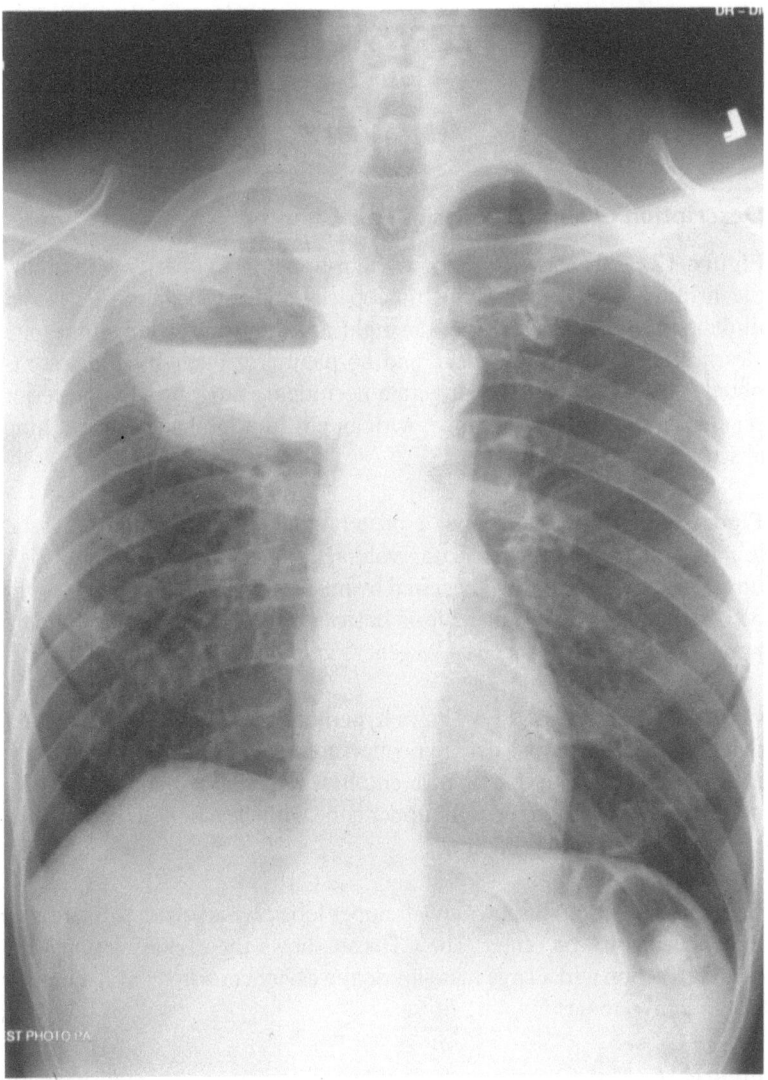

Fig. 17

Cavitary Lesions

Answers

Description of Chest X-rays in This Chapter

Figure 12. This chest x-ray shows right upper zone opacity with multiple air-fluid levels. Surrounding this opacity and the air-fluid levels is an ill-defined infiltrate. Note that the right apex and lower lung zones are clear. The left lung is also clear, and no pleural or mediastinal disease is noted. This x-ray is consistent with a necrotizing process in the posterior segment of the right upper lobe, with an air-fluid level such as in a lung abscess.

Figure 13. This CXR shows a bilateral process with multiple cystic lesions primarily on the left. Lung volumes appear small and there is left upper zone cicatrization as suggested by hilar retraction. This picture could be consistent with old tuberculosis but can also be seen in a necrotizing granulomatous disease such as Wegener's granulomatosis.

Figure 14. This chest x-ray shows hyperlucent lung fields with flattened diaphragm. Areas of vascular attenuation are noted especially in the upper zones, consistent with central lobar emphysema. A 3.5 × 3-cm circular cavitary shadow is seen in the right upper zone with elevation of the horizontal fissure and the right hilum.

Figure 15. This CXR shows an left upper lobe cavitary mass with areas of hyperlucency in the center. The CT scan shows the cavitary lesion with pleural reaction and a large mass inside the cavity consistent with a fungus ball or a mycetoma.

Figure 16. This CXR shows areas of hyperlucency on the right side with decreased vascular markings. On the left, the lung volume appears small with nodular infiltrates with some areas of confluence in the left middle zone. A large cavitary lesion is seen in the left upper lobe with signs of volume loss and tracheal shift.

Figure 17. This PA and lateral chest x-ray shows a large right upper lobe mass with an air-fluid level. This mass has a very thick wall with irregular inner margins and is abutting the mediastinum. Differential diagnosis in this case would include lung abscess or cavitary squamous cell carcinoma.

General Discussion

The x-ray differential for infiltrates with areas of breakdown or cavitation and signs of loss of volume or retraction includes primarily inflammatory diseases such as TB, sarcoidosis, nontuberculous mycobacterial diseases (MOTT/NTM), nocardia, fungal diseases, and gram-negative necrotizing pneumonia. Postobstructive pneumonia secondary to tumor or foreign body may cavitate and cause volume loss. Cavitary cancer usually does not retract lung tissue but may push adjacent structures. An "air-crescent sign" on a chest x-ray or a "halo sign" on CT scan suggests a fungus ball in a patient with underlying bullous/fibrotic/cavitary disease. Clinical hints that may be helpful include clubbing that may suggest lung abscess or a cavitary carcinoma and fluctuating fluid level suggesting instability due to infection or ongoing hemoptysis. Associated nasal symptoms may suggest Wegener's granulomatosis.

Specific Discussion

19–20. The answers are 19-c, 20-a. The presence of a subacute illness with foul-smelling sputum and clubbing is a classical presentation for a lung abscess, which is caused by mixed aerobic and anaerobic infection. Pneumococcal pneumonia generally does not produce a necrotizing picture, and PCP in an immune-compromised patient usually appears as a diffuse reticular pattern, but cystic and cavitary areas may be present. A lung abscess represents a localized area of lung necrosis with a thick wall and an acute angle to the chest wall. An air-fluid level is seen, representing a communication with the bronchial tree. The fluid level diameter is usually similar on PA and lateral chest films with a lung abscess and is often considerably different with empyema. Differentiation between an empyema and a lung abscess is crucial since the former requires tube thoracostomy, while the latter is adequately treated with antibiotics and postural drainage. Immediate bronchoscopy may not be needed unless an endobronchial obstruction is suspected or there is a history of choking or aspiration. Contrast CT scans may be helpful to see the split pleural sign with marked visceral and parietal pleural thickening in an empyema.

21–22. The answers are 21-b, 22-b. Nasal symptoms with a nodular/cavitary process on the chest x-ray are suggestive of Wegener's granulomatosis. This is most often associated with a positive C-ANCA. Other options mentioned are not seen in this condition.

23. The answer is b. An upper lobe cavitary lesion in a patient with underlying COPD suggests TB or NTM (MOTT). AFB-positive smears may culture out *Mycobacterium kansasii* or *M. avium-intracellulare* complex (MAC). Another possibility is nocardia infection. Actinomyces can present as upper lobe cavitary disease but is not acid-fast-positive on smear and is commonly seen with skin infection and fistula formation. The diagnosis of *M. avium* disease (MAC) is established by fulfilling clinical radiographic and culture criteria. The diagnosis should be suspected with symptoms of cough, fever, and weight loss with progressive infiltrates, cavitation, and multiple nodules. Patients without underlying lung disease who have chronic pulmonary infections are predominantly women and nonsmokers. High-resolution CT scan typically shows multiple small nodules with bronchiectasis. The diagnosis must be established bacteriologically since some nontuberculous mycobacteria are commonly found in nature and contamination of specimen can occur. Therefore, the diagnosis of MOTT pulmonary disease requires the following: three positive cultures with negative AFP smears; two positive cultures and one positive smear; a single bronchial specimen with a positive culture of 2 to 4+ growth; a positive AFB smear and a positive culture of any biopsy specimen; granuloma by biopsy with one positive culture from any respiratory specimen; or a growth of MAC from any usually sterile extrapulmonary site. Although transient infection with spontaneous resolution occurs, significant growth on culture means disease is present. Mycobacterial disease due to nontuberculous mycobacteria is now more common than tuberculosis in the United States. It is generally prevalent in specific areas such as the Southeast and the Gulf Coast region. According to the CDC, one-third to one-fourth of all isolates of mycobacteria are due to nontuberculous mycobacteria. Natural waters appear to be the likely environmental source of these organisms, which can be isolated from tap water or even hospital water. Person-to-person transmission is thought to be unlikely. Clinical syndromes of MAI disease in nonimmune non-HIV individuals occur in older patients, particularly smokers and alcoholics with COPD. These syndromes may present as upper lobe infiltrates or cavitary or solitary nodules.

Patients can develop chronic bronchiectasis or cystic fibrosis. In nonsmoking women older than 50, multiple small and medium-sized nodules may be seen. Upper lobe or lingular infiltrates have been described. Coughing and purulent sputum for an average of 6 mo may be present.

24–25. The answers are 24-d, 25-d. The clinical and radiological scenario suggests a mycetoma in a patient with underlying sarcoidosis. The presentations of aspergillus-related disease in the lung include allergic alveolitis, invasive microangiopathic aspergillosis, allergic bronchopulmonary aspergillosis (ABPA) in an asthmatic, or a fungus ball, as seen in this patient. Colonization may also occur, and culture contamination is possible since the organism is ubiquitous. Hemoptysis can be very severe in cases of aspergilloma and requires invasive or semi-invasive interventions. Bronchial artery embolization is most helpful in controlling symptoms in patients who are poor surgical candidates for resection of the affected lobe. However, recurrent hemoptysis is common. The aspergilloma may wax and wane in size and even spontaneously disappear.

Aspergillosis in the lung can present in a variety of other ways. Mucoid impaction can be a manifestation of ABPA. Mucoid impactions can occur in chronic asthma, chronic bronchitis, and cystic fibrosis, as well as behind central obstructions such as bronchial carcinoid and bronchial atresia. Invasive aspergillosis is usually seen in immune-compromised patients or following prolonged neutropenia. A characteristic radiograph described as a nodule with an "air-crescent sign" is seen in bone marrow transplant patients usually following return of the neutrophil count. Allergic bronchopulmonary aspergillosis is a hypersensitivity disease due to aspergillosis antigens associated with mucus plugs that are colonized with aspergillosis species. ABPA is caused by an immune reaction to aspergillosis fungus—usually fumigatus, although it can be seen in other mycoses. Radiographic features include fleeting infiltrates representing eosonophilic pneumonia, mucoid infection or atelectasis, and proximal or central bronchiectasis with a finger-and-glove pattern. Typically, there is little tissue invasion associated with ABPA, but organisms may be found adjacent to the walls. ABPA usually develops in patients with a history of longstanding asthma. In the acute phase, common findings include type I and type III hypersensitivity reactions. Reaction to aspergillosis antigens and peripheral and sputum eosinophilia is seen. Positive IgE, IG, and IA antibodies against the specific organisms with the marked elevation of IE level up to

1000 IU is characteristic. An increase in IE precedes radiographic findings and is usually a good index of disease activity. A normal IE in a patient with suspected ABPA virtually rules out the diagnosis. ABPA can be classified into stages. Stage 1 is acute, in which treatment with corticosteroids assures dramatic improvement. Stage II is remission, which may last for months or years. Stage III is recurrent exacerbation characterized by acute-phase symptoms with total IE almost doubling. Stage IV is defined as patients requiring continuous corticosteroids. Stage V is end-stage fibrotic lung disease. As a clinical follow-up, serial IgE testing every 3 mo is advisable. Aspergillosis may be sporadically isolated from sputum culture, but this is not necessary for diagnosis.

26–27. The answers are 26-a, 27-b. This clinical and radiographic presentation is seen in TB. Four-drug anti-TB treatment should be promptly started based on this clinical and radiological suspicion. There is no role for single-drug chemoprophylaxis in this case. ACE levels are of some prognostic value in sarcoidosis. Starting empirical antifungal treatment would be inappropriate in this clinical context.

28–29. The answers are 28-b, 29-d. The clinical history suggests a chronic illness with stigmata of an underlying malignancy. A large, thick-walled abscess formation may be seen secondary to a postobstructive pneumonia. Bronchoscopy is helpful to see if there is a lesion causing this obstruction and is the appropriate next step.

Hyperlucent Lung

DIRECTIONS: Each item below contains a question or incomplete statement followed by suggested responses. Select the **one best** response to each question.

Items 30–31

A 50-year-old male smoker is evaluated for chronic shortness of breath. On physical examination his vital signs are: pulse 110 bpm; temperature normal; respirations 30/min with use of accessory muscles and pursed-lip breathing; blood pressure 110/78 mm Hg. Other pertinent findings are: heart exam: apex beat (impulse) is medial to the midclavicular line with generalized decreased breath sounds on lung exam; ABGs (Fio_2 0.21): pH 7.38; Pco_2 47 mm Hg; Po_2 67 mm Hg. PFTs/spirometry: FVC 2.80 L (67% of predicted); FEV$_1$ 1.56 (50% of predicted); FEV$_1$/FVC% 56%; TLC 134% of predicted; RV 170% of predicted; DLCO 43% of predicted. There is no reversibility with bronchodilators. Chest radiographs are shown below in Fig. 18.

30. What is the most likely diagnosis?

a. Bronchial asthma with status asthmaticus
b. Emphysema
c. Chronic bronchitis
d. Tuberous sclerosis

31. Associated with the above condition is

a. Obstructive sleep apnea
b. Increased IgE levels
c. Respiratory failure with increased A-aDo_2 gradient
d. Clubbing

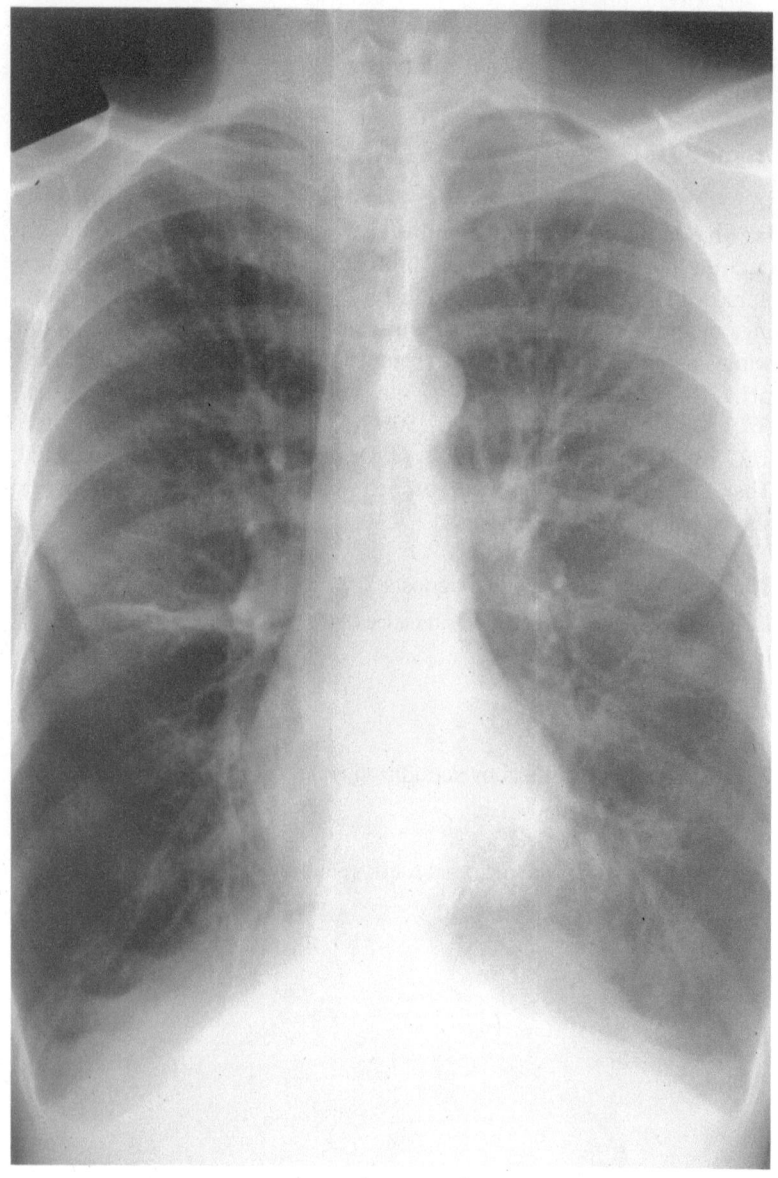

Fig. 18a

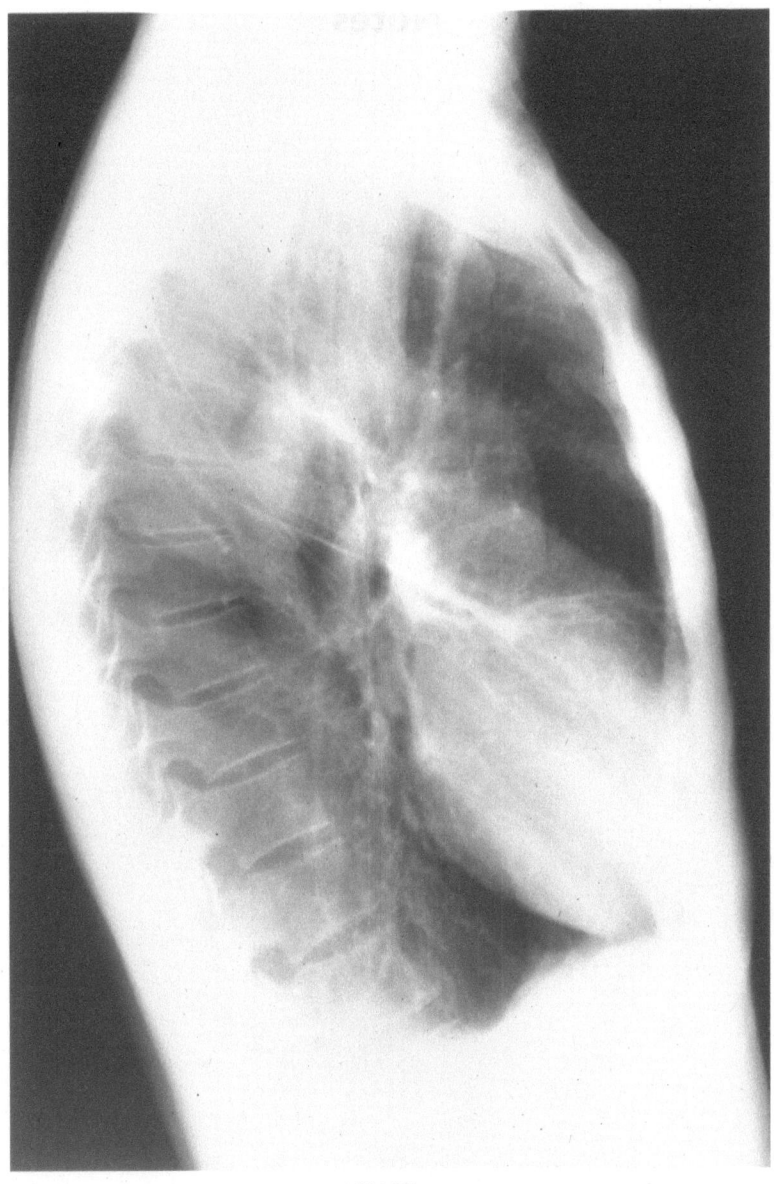

Fig. 18b

Notes

Items 32–33

A 38-year-old man is admitted with progressive shortness of breath and cough. He denies any fever, chills, or purulent sputum production. He wants to be evaluated to determine the reasons for his symptoms. On exam, he is afebrile and has decreased breath sounds with hyperresonant upper lung field more obvious on the right. ABGs on RA: pH 7.35; P_{CO_2} 38 mm Hg; P_{O_2} 78 mm Hg. Spirometry: FVC 1.72 (70% of predicted); FEV_1 1.34 L (60% of predicted); FEV_1/FVC% 76%; TLC 4.1 L (100% of predicted); TLC by helium dilution method 3.4 (71%); DLCO 70% of predicted. There is no bronchodilator response. Chest radiographs are shown below in Fig. 19.

32. What is the most likely diagnosis?

a. Severe emphysema
b. Bulla
c. Pneumothorax
d. Bronchiectasis

33. What is the next management option?

a. Place a chest tube urgently
b. Increase bronchodilator dosage and frequency
c. Start chest physical therapy
d. Perform CT scan of chest

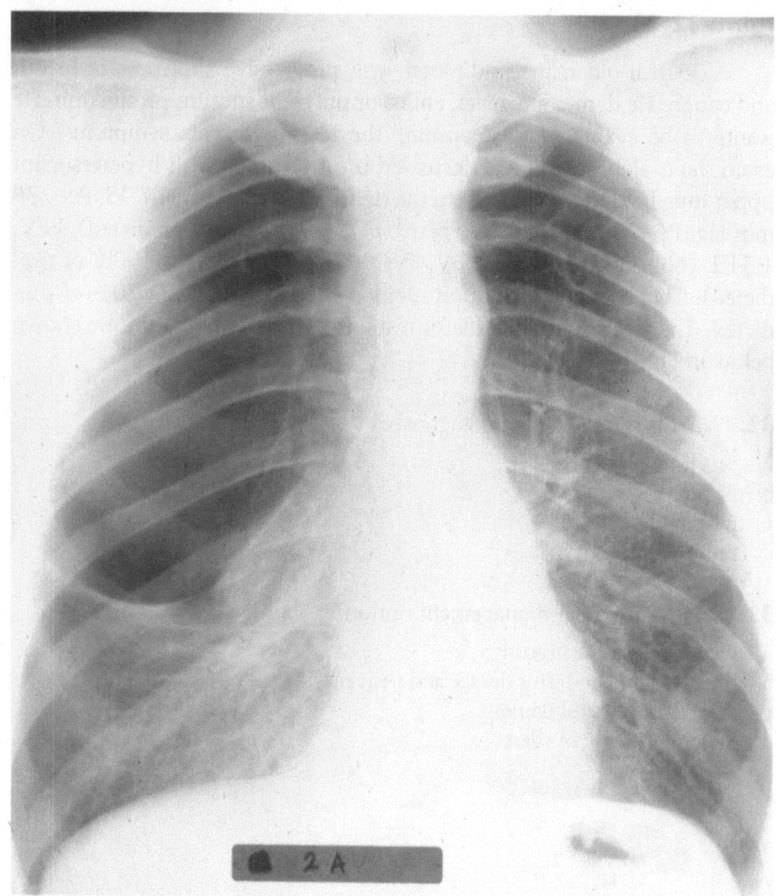

Fig. 19a

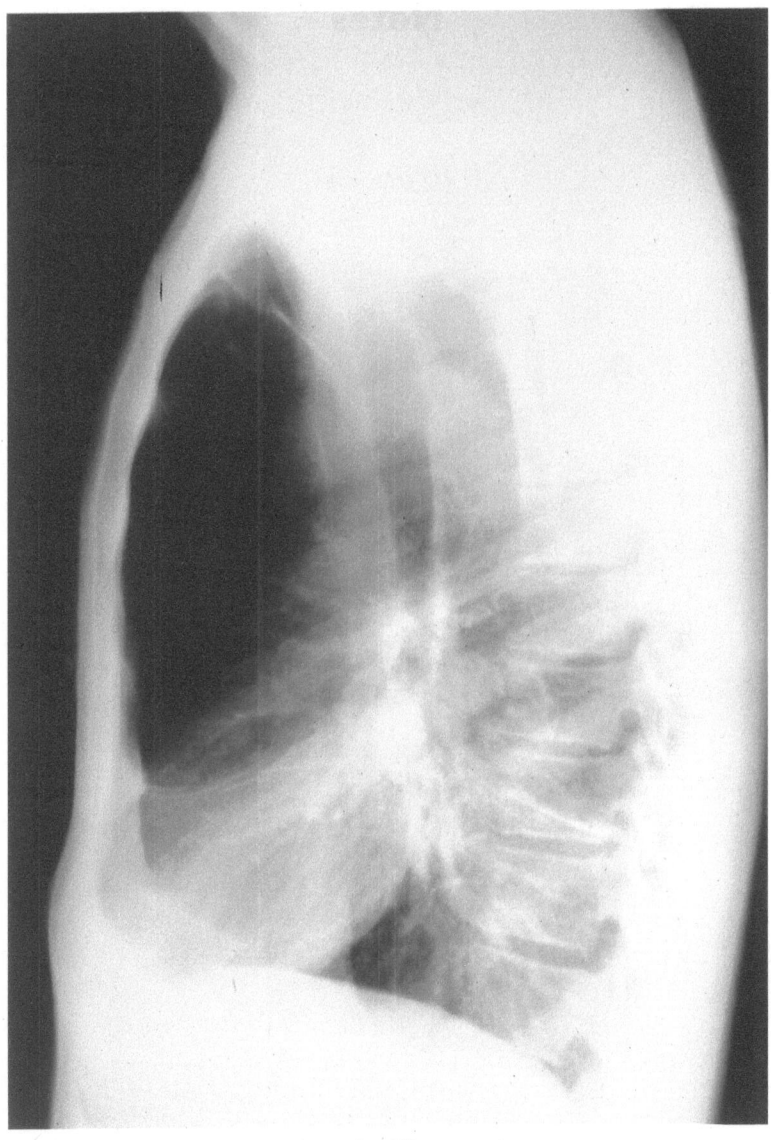

Fig. 19b

Notes

Items 34–35

A 39-year-old man, a smoker since age 16, is seen in the clinic with complaints of fever, cough, and production of yellowish sputum. He has been chronically short of breath, but these symptoms have increased over the last week after he developed a flulike illness. On exam, he is febrile and looks ill. Lung exam reveals diffuse wheezing with egophony and whispering pectoriloquy on the right side. ABGs show PO_2 of 55 mm Hg on room air, and sputum is negative for TB. Chest x-rays are shown in Fig. 20.

34. The next step in the management of this patient would be

a. Arrange with intervention radiology to do a needle aspiration
b. Consult thoracic surgery for lung reduction surgery
c. Start antibiotic and O_2 therapy
d. Admit patient in an isolation room

35. Appropriate measures at the first follow-up should include

a. Pneumococcal and influenza vaccine
b. Allergy testing
c. Detailed occupational history
d. Genetic counseling

68 Chest Radiology

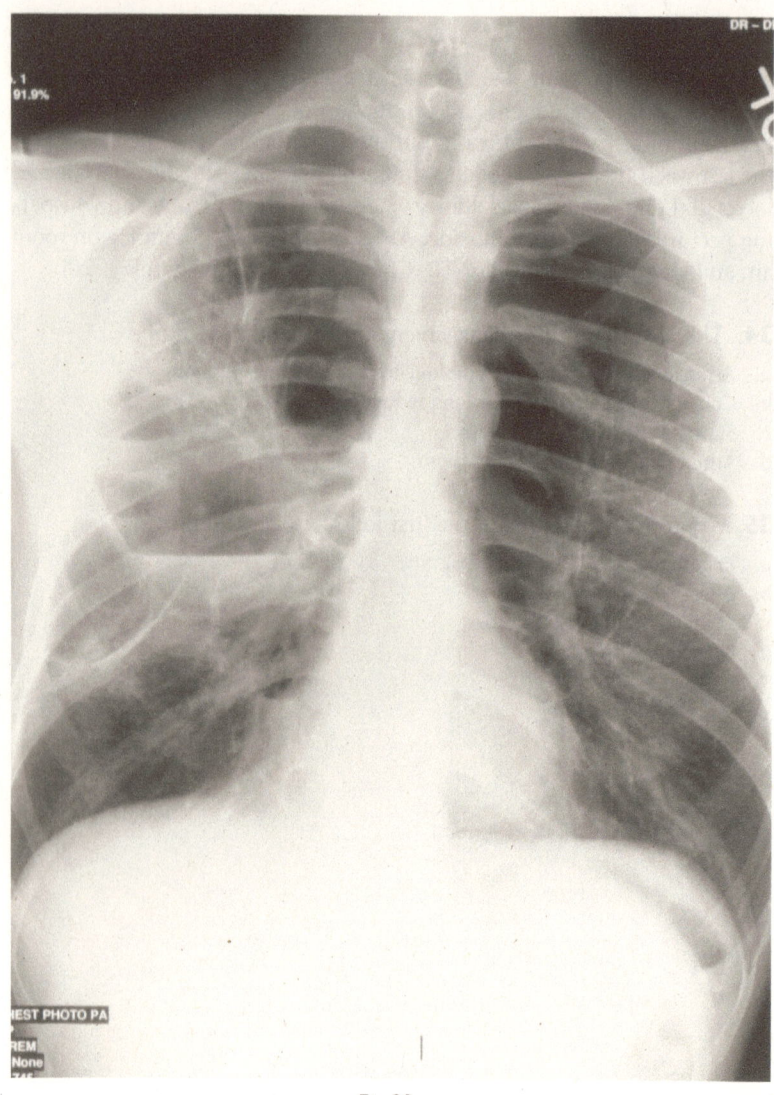

Fig. 20a

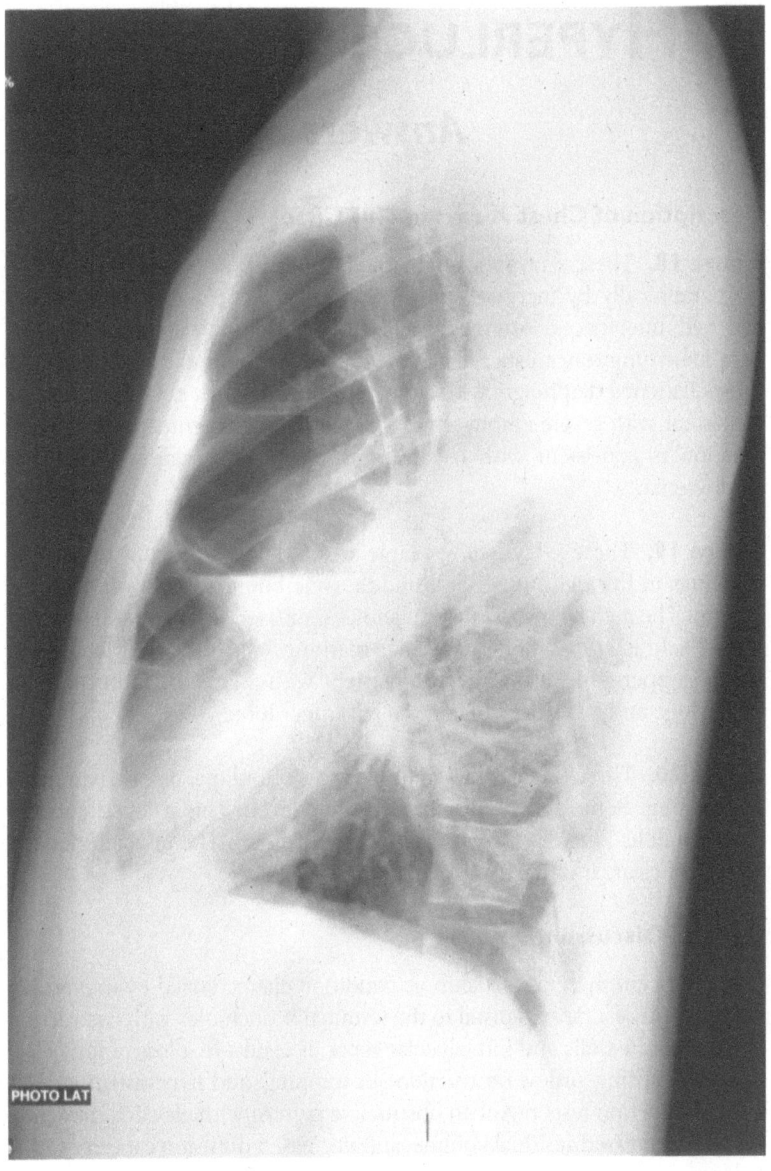

Fig. 20b

Hyperlucent Lung

Answers

Description of Chest X-rays in This Chapter

Figure 18. These x-rays show a marked degree of hyperinflation depicted radiographically by increased lung volume with flattened diaphragm and widened interspaces. Attenuation of the pulmonary vasculature in the peripheral lung zones, especially in the lower zones, is seen. The lateral CXR shows flattened diaphragm with large retrosternal airspace. These x-rays are consistent with severe emphysema. The lower lobe accentuation of hyperinflation is consistent with α_1 antitrypsin deficiency causing panacinar emphysema.

Figure 19. These x-rays show a large area of hyperlucency with no lung markings in the right upper and middle zone bounded by a very distinct margin. The area below the margin shows increased density and compression. There is attenuation of vascular markings and increased lucency in the left upper zone also. This is consistent with a large bulla in the right upper lobe and a smaller bulla in the left upper lobe.

Figure 20. These x-rays show multiple areas of bullous disease with hairline margins. Some of the bullae have air-fluid levels. This is consistent with severe bullous lung disease with secondary infection. The upper zones and apices are clear, and this study is not typical of TB.

General Discussion

Pulmonary emphysema is a chronic condition characterized by irreversible enlargement of airspaces distal to the terminal bronchioles with destruction of the alveolar walls and intraalveolar septa. It results in a loss of lung elastic recoil causing airflow obstruction, air trapping, and hyperinflation. Pulmonary function tests reveal an obstructive pattern with elevated total lung capacity, increased residual volume, and decreased diffusion capacity. Chest x-ray reveals all signs of hyperinflation as illustrated above. A bulla is an air-containing space larger than 1 cm in the lung parenchyma generally representing focal emphysema. Blebs are smaller airspaces occurring within the subpleural or pleural layers. A cyst is a rounded airspace with a well-defined wall consisting of epithelium or fibrous tissue containing air, but not necessarily associated with emphysema. Cysts may contain varying amounts of fluid due to epithelial fluid secretion associated with cystic or paracystic infection or tumor.

Specific Discussion

30–31. The answers are 30-b, 31-c. The physical signs and CXR suggest emphysema. This is confirmed by an obstructive ventilatory impairment with hyperinflation, air trapping, and reduced diffusion. In bronchial asthma, there would typically be marked bronchodilator response, and the patient with chronic bronchitis would present with chronic sputum production. Tuberous sclerosis presents radiographically as hyperinflation and lower zone infiltrates, but clinically is a systemic disease with a clinical triad of mental retardation, seizure disorder, and dermal angiofibromas called adenoma sebaceum. Pulmonary disease is rare (it is seen in less than 1% of cases) and presents with pneumothoraces and hemoptysis. In this case with emphysema, complications include respiratory failure. Increased IgE levels are associated with allergic bronchial asthma; obstructive sleep apnea and clubbing do not have an increased association with this condition. CT scan is the most sensitive imaging modality to reliably detect emphysema. Although pulmonary artery enlargement and mild pulmonary arterial hypertension are common in advanced emphysema, radiographic evaluation of pulmonary artery size is a poor indicator of PA pressures. Other concomitant pulmonary disease processes such as pneumonia or pulmonary edema may present in an atypical fashion in a patient with emphysema. Forms of emphysema include the following:

1. *Centrilobular emphysema* is the most common form, found predominantly in cigarette smokers. The destructive process begins with involvement of the center of the secondary lobule and extends into the lung parenchyma. The upper lobes are more frequently involved.
2. *Panacinar emphysema* begins with the involvement of the entire secondary lobule with diffuse, widespread lung destruction. It is seen in α_1 antitrypsin deficiency and has lower zone predominance.
3. *Paraseptal emphysema* refers to peripheral lung destruction adjacent to the visceral pleura and interlobular septa. Progressive dyspnea associ-

ated with increasing paraseptal emphysema forming bullae refers to the "vanishing lung syndrome" (see below).
4. *Congenital emphysema* is seen in the first few months of life and refers to a large hyperlucent lobe associated with compressive and mass effect on the adjacent structures.
5. *Compensatory emphysema* refers to hyperlucent and hyperinflated airspaces adjacent to areas of deformity, atelectasis, or resection of lung and represents overexpansion without actual lung destruction.
6. *Scar emphysema* is associated with conditions of fibrosis and scarring and associated honeycombing as in stage 4 sarcoidosis or chronic inflammatory conditions.

32–33. The answers are 32-b, 33-d. The CXR shows a large bulla, which accounts for the symptoms of this patient. Discrepancy in total lung capacity as assessed by the helium dilution and body plethysmography methods suggests significant gas trapping in the bulla and can be used to estimate the volume of the bulla. Bullae become symptomatic as they enlarge, and the goal of surgical therapy is to excise them to enable the surrounding tissue to reexpand. CT scan is helpful to determine the size, extent, and number of bullae present. It also helps in evaluating the anatomy of the remaining lung and its potential for effective reexpansion. PFTs may show a restrictive pattern if the bulla does not communicate with the airways. If there is no diffuse, widespread emphysema and profound hypoxemia or hypercarbia is not present, surgical resection of the bulla is likely to improve the symptoms. Placement of a chest tube in this case would convert an intrapulmonary closed airspace into a bronchopleural cutaneous fistula and is therefore not an appropriate option.

34–35. The answers are 34-c, 35-a. One of the complications of multiple air-containing cystic spaces or bullae is infection, especially if open communication with airways is present. This is seen as multiple air-fluid levels, the immediate treatment plan should include aggressive antibiotic therapy and oxygen supplementation. Other options are inappropriate at this stage. As sputum is negative for AFB, respiratory isolation is not necessary. Needle aspiration in severe bullous disease is hazardous, and lung reduction surgery may be a long-term option but is clearly not indicated during acute infection. As a follow-up, prevention of pneumonia and influenza is of top priority because it has been shown to reduce mortality and morbidity. Other options outlined serve no specific purpose.

Cysts and Cystic-Appearing Lesions

DIRECTIONS: Each item below contains a question or incomplete statement followed by suggested responses. Select the **one best** response to each question.

Items 36–37

A 31-year-old African American man is admitted with increasing cough, fever, and sputum production. He gives a history of repeated infections and "pneumonias" since childhood. Lung exam reveals diffuse rhonchi and bilateral crackles, more so in the left lung field. Routine labs are normal except for a polymorphonuclear leukocytosis. Chest radiograph is shown below in Fig. 21.

36. What is the most likely diagnosis?
a. Bronchiectasis
b. Cystic fibrosis
c. Sarcoidosis
d. Allergic bronchopulmonary aspergillosis

37. What is the next management option?
a. Bronchoscopy
b. Steroid Rx
c. Antibiotics and postural drainage
d. Surgical consult

Cysts and Cystic-Appearing Lesions 75

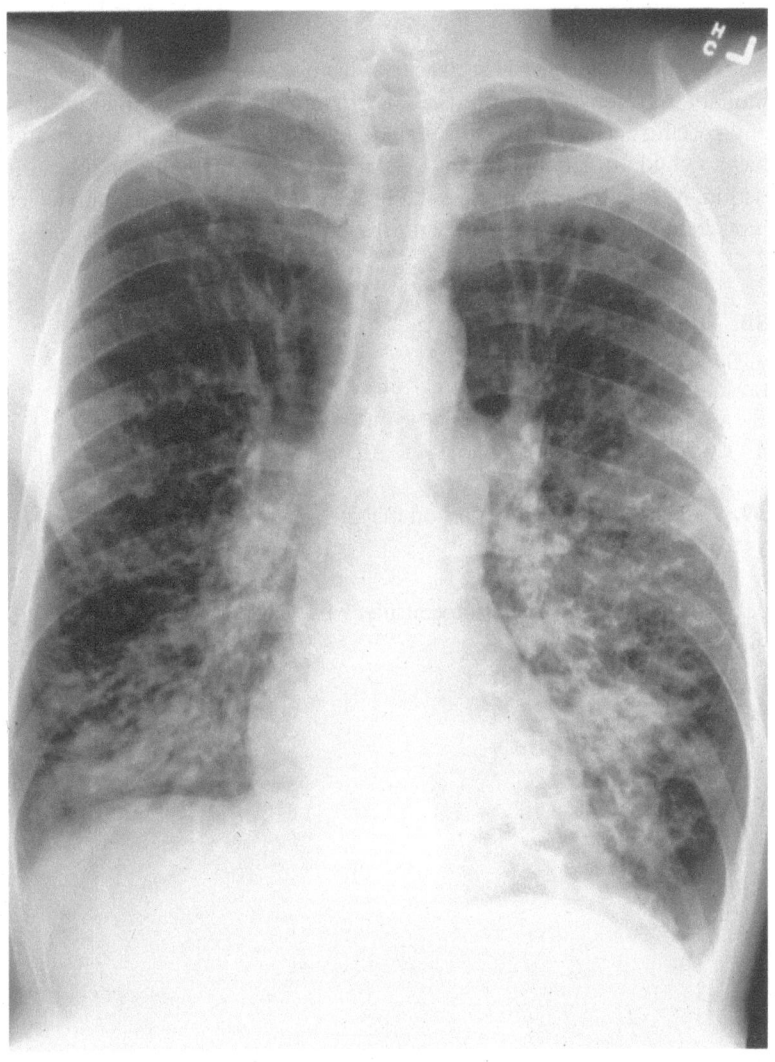

Fig. 21

Items 38-39

A 27-year-old man is seen with a history of chronic sinus and pulmonary infections. He works as a salesperson in a retail outlet and denies any specific occupational exposure. He lives with his wife of 4 years and has no children. Family and travel history is noncontributory. On examination, he is in no acute distress. Lung exam reveals crackles in both lower lung zones and extremities show no clubbing. CXR is shown below in Fig. 22.

38. The most likely diagnosis is
a. IgA deficiency
b. Kartagener syndrome
c. Aspiration pneumonia
d. Cystic fibrosis

39. Associated with this condition may be
a. Reflux esophagitis
b. Absent frontal sinuses
c. Methicillin-resistant staphylococcal infection
d. Positive ANA

Cysts and Cystic-Appearing Lesions 77

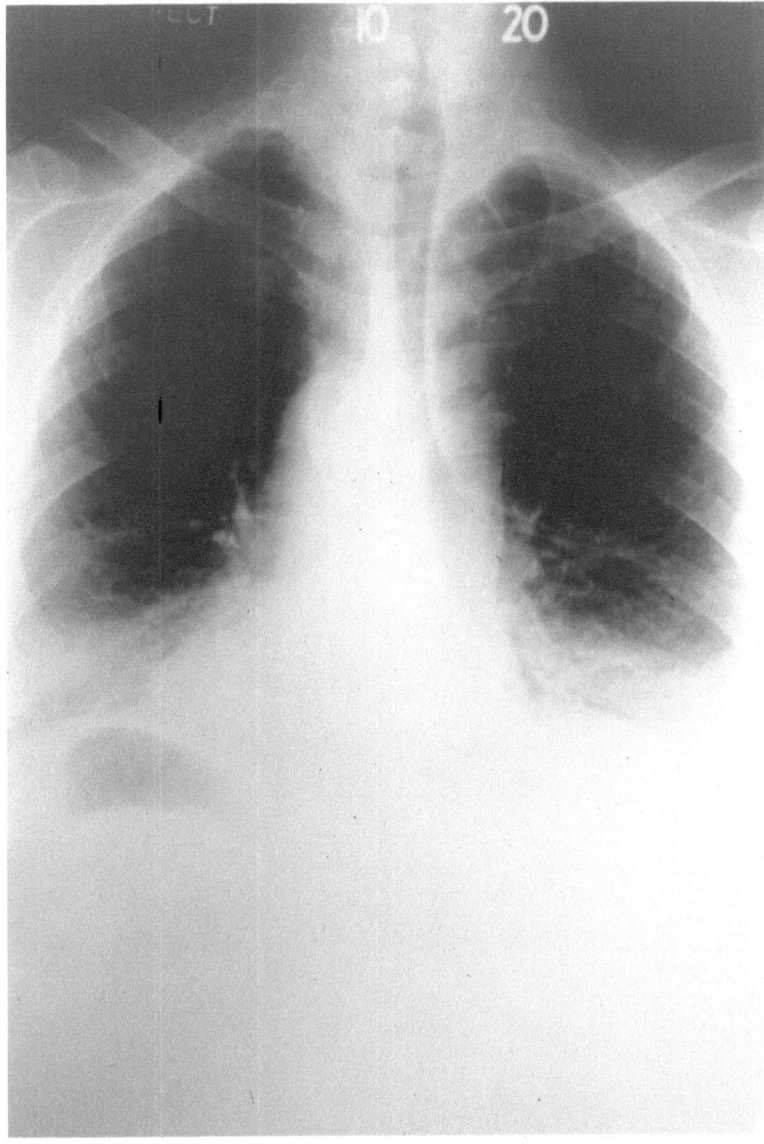

Fig. 22

40. A 29-year-old woman is referred to the clinic with a history of repeated respiratory tract infections. There is no significant travel history and she denies any possibility of foreign body aspiration. On examination, she has coarse crackles in the left lower lung zone. CXR is shown in Fig. 23. Based on the history and CXR, the next diagnostic step should be

a. Contrast CT scan of the chest and upper abdomen
b. Bronchogram
c. Bronchoscopy
d. Determination of serum immunoglobulin levels

Cysts and Cystic-Appearing Lesions 79

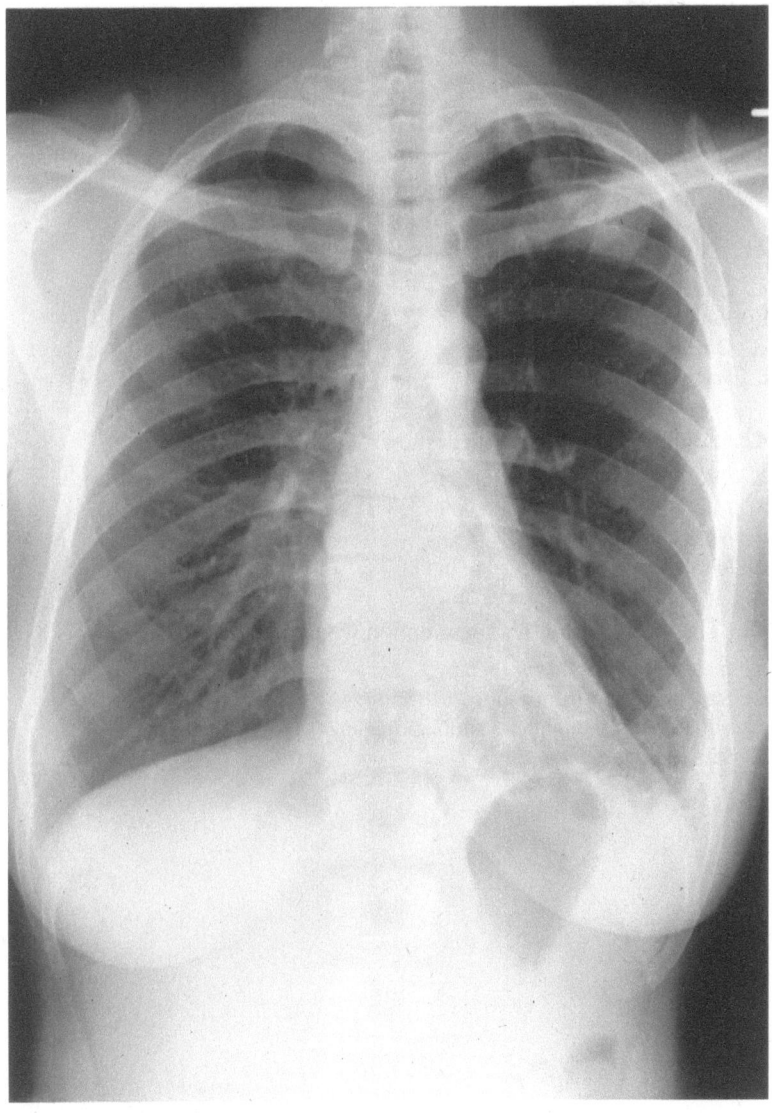

Fig. 23

Items 41–43

A 24-year-old male law student presents with a 3-wk history of increasing dyspnea. He has a history of chronic sputum production of about 100 cc of purulent material each day for many years. In the past, he was hospitalized for a left pneumothorax. He is on inhaled bronchodilator as an outpatient. CXR is shown below in Fig. 24.

41. Physical exam will most likely show
a. Clubbing
b. Koilonychia
c. Oncholysis
d. Pectus excavatum

42. Spirometry will most likely show
a. FVC 60%; FEV_1 40%; ratio 66%
b. FVC 60%; FEV_1 62%; ratio 90%
c. Normal
d. Normal except mild decrease in FEF_{25-75}

43. The most helpful treatment option would be
a. Increase bronchodilator therapy
b. Start broad-spectrum antibiotic therapy
c. Initiate anti-pseudomonas antibiotic regimen
d. Start oral steroids

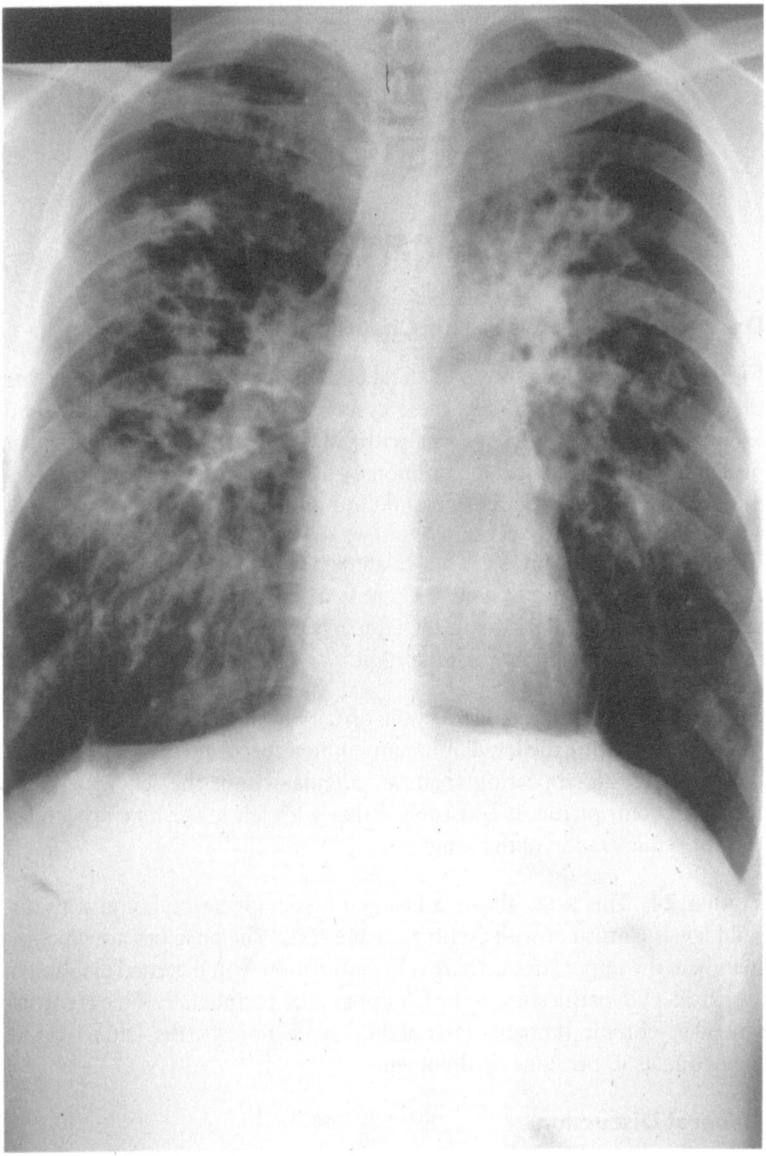

Cysts and Cystic-Appearing Lesions

Fig. 24

CYSTS AND CYSTIC-APPEARING LESIONS

Answers

Description of X-rays in This Chapter

Figure 21. This x-ray shows bilateral cystic-appearing opacities involving the lower and middle zones. These cysts have distinct walls and air-fluid levels. This picture is consistent with bilateral lower lobe and lingular bronchiectasis. Note the large pulmonary arteries, which may suggest secondary pulmonary hypertension and cor pulmonale.

Figure 22. This x-ray shows a bilateral lower zone hazy density with small cystic-appearing shadows. There is dextrocardia with situs inversus totalis, i.e., a right aortic arch, the stomach bubble on the right side, and the left diaphragm higher than the right.

Figure 23. This x-ray shows a cystic opacity in the left lower lobe behind the heart obscuring the left diaphragm but not obscuring the left heart border. These cystic-appearing shadows originate from the left lower lobe bronchus. This picture is consistent either with left lower lobe bronchiectasis or sequestration of the lung.

Figure 24. This x-ray shows a bilateral cystic-appearing lesion with air-fluid levels consistent with cystic bronchiectasis. The opacities are predominantly in the upper zones. There is hyperinflation with flattened diaphragm and areas of hyperlucency in the left upper lobe peripherally. This is consistent with chronic bronchiectasis and/or cystic fibrosis; the latter is more likely due its upper zone predominance.

General Discussion

Bronchiectasis refers to an irreversible bronchial dilatation with bronchial wall thickening as a result of infection and inflammation. It can be congenital, as seen in cystic fibrosis and immotile cilia syndromes. Symptoms include chronic recurrent cough, sputum production, and hemoptysis. Life-threatening hemoptysis can occur. Conditions associated with bronchiectasis include airway obstruction, foreign body impaction, chronic airway or inhalational injury, allergic bronchopulmonary aspergillosis/mycosis (ABPA/ABPM), cystic fibrosis, and ciliary dyskinesia/immotile cilia syndromes, recurrent aspiration, and idiopathic bronchiectasis. Focal bronchiectasis can also result from bronchial stenosis with occlusion due an endobronchial lesion with mucoid infection or as a result of a prior severe pneumonia. Impaired mucociliary clearance and hypogammaglobulinemia have lower lobe predominance. Cystic fibrosis has upper lobe predominance, whereas bronchiectasis associated with ABPA is central in location. Bronchiectasis is often classified as cylindrical, varicose, saccular/cystic, or traction. Cylindrical or tubular bronchiectasis is due to uniform fusiform dilation and is seen as "tram-track" lines on x-ray. Varicose bronchiectasis appears as beaded with alternating areas of dilatation and constriction as seen in cystic fibrosis. Saccular or cystic bronchiectasis is manifested by marked bronchial dilation with peripheral ballooning of the cystic spaces and air-fluid levels and is often associated with bronchial stenosis. Traction bronchiectasis is the result of fibrotic distortion of the lung caused by infection, radiation, or end-stage lung disease, and is seen most commonly in the lung periphery.

Specific Discussion

36–37. The answers are 36-a, 37-c. The history is suggestive of bronchiectasis, and the bilateral cystic-appearing lesions on the CXR are consistent with that diagnosis. Cystic fibrosis is generally predominant in the upper zone. Sarcoidosis rarely presents with this history, and the fibrotic changes in sarcoidosis are usually in the upper lobes. Allergic bronchopulmonary aspergillosis is seen with an underlying asthmatic condition. The next management option would be to give antibiotics and intensify postural drainage. Steroids would only be indicated if there is severe respiratory failure and bronchospasm. Bronchoscopy and surgical consult are inappropriate options at this stage.

38–39. The answers are 38-b, 39-b. The chest x-ray shows dextrocardia and bilateral bronchiectasis as seen in immotile cilia syndrome. Kartagener syndrome is the immotile cilia syndrome with situs inversus totalis.

This is an autosomal recessive disease characterized by structural and functional abnormalities of the cilia resulting in impaired mucus clearance, recurrent infection, chronic sinobronchial infections, and infertility. Frontal sinuses are often absent or hypoplastic. Chronic mucus impaction and infections lead to bronchiectasis.

40. The answer is a. The chest x-ray and clinical history suggest bronchiectasis of the left lower lobe. Bronchograms are not done anymore because of frequent complications and the fact that a CT scan can confirm the diagnosis. Bronchoscopy would not reveal any additional information unless there is a history of foreign body aspiration. Determination of immunoglobulin levels would be helpful in a patient with chronic generalized or multilobar infection or frequent skin infections. The differential diagnosis in this case would include pulmonary sequestration, which could present with a similar radiological picture. A pulmonary sequestration is an abnormal embryonic lung tissue that is segregated from the tracheal bronchial system and does not communicate through normal bronchus. Since the sequestrated lung is cystic, it does not function normally. There are two types of pulmonary sequestration. Intralobar sequestrations, seen most frequently in adults, are located within the visceral pleura and are contained within the lung parenchyma. Extralobar sequestrations, which are located outside the visceral pleura, have their own separate pleural covering. The most common location for intralobar sequestration is the posterior basilar segments of the lower lobe. It is characterized by bronchiectasis with cystic areas containing mucus or mucopurulent material, and is lined with ciliated columnar or cuboidal epithelium. The walls may contain cartilage and glands. In the adult, multifocal epithelial changes can occur, and dysplastic or carcinomatotic changes have been reported within intralobar sequestrations. The most common site of the region of the anomalous arterial supply in pulmonary sequestration is the thoracic aorta, followed by the abdominal aorta and intercostal arteries. Cough and hemoptysis may be the initial symptoms. On plain x-ray, intralobar sequestration appears as a solid or cystic mass located in the lower lobe. Air-fluid levels are seen and may be mistaken for pneumonia, bronchiectasis, or abscess formation. Bronchoscopy reveals no abnormality, and for a definitive diagnosis of sequestration it is important to demonstrate the systemic arterial supply. CT scan or aortography can accomplish this. Untreated sequestration has an associated morbidity related to infection, vascular shunting and hemoptysis; thus, resection is the treatment of choice.

41–43. The answers are 41-a, 42-a, 43-c. The history and chest x-ray are consistent with cystic fibrosis with bilateral cystic upper zone predominance. Physical exam would reveal clubbing; spirometry would show a mixed obstructive with restrictive picture. The best option would be to initiate anti-pseudomonas antibiotics. Cystic fibrosis is an autosomal recessive disease characterized by exocrine gland dysfunction with viscous secretions. It is the most common inherited lung disease in whites with associated gene mutation. Diagnosis is usually based on clinical presentation and excessive chloride secretion in the sweat glands. Pulmonary manifestations include recurrent pneumonia with mucus plugging and increased morbidity and mortality due to staphylococcal and pseudomonas infection. Complications may include pneumothorax, rupture of a subpleural bleb, hemoptysis, lung abscesses, and empyema. Massive hemoptysis and cor pulmonale may cause respiratory failure and increase mortality.

Diffuse Interstitial Disease

DIRECTIONS: Each item below contains a question or incomplete statement followed by suggested responses. Select the **one best** response to each question.

Items 44–46

A 49-year-old white woman presents with progressive cough and dyspnea. She denies any history of arthritis, skin lesions, or eye complaints. On physical examination, vital signs are: pulse 90 bpm; temperature 98°F; respirations 32/min; blood pressure 119/76 mm Hg. General exam: patient is in moderate distress, and pertinent physical findings reveal clubbing of the fingers and bilateral "Velcro" rales on lung auscultation. ABGs on room air: pH 7.47; P_{CO_2} 32 mm Hg; P_{O_2} 60 mm Hg with further desaturation on mild exertion. Chest radiograph is shown below in Fig. 25.

44. Least likely to be associated with this condition is
a. Positive antinuclear antigen
b. Positive rheumatoid factor
c. Increased erythrocyte sedimentation rate
d. Increased IgE

45. What is the most likely diagnosis?
a. Idiopathic pulmonary fibrosis
b. Langerhans granulomatosis/histiocytosis-X disorders
c. Rheumatoid lung
d. Sarcoidosis

46. PFTS would be expected to show
a. An obstructive pattern
b. A restrictive pattern
c. A normal pattern
d. A reversible obstructive pattern

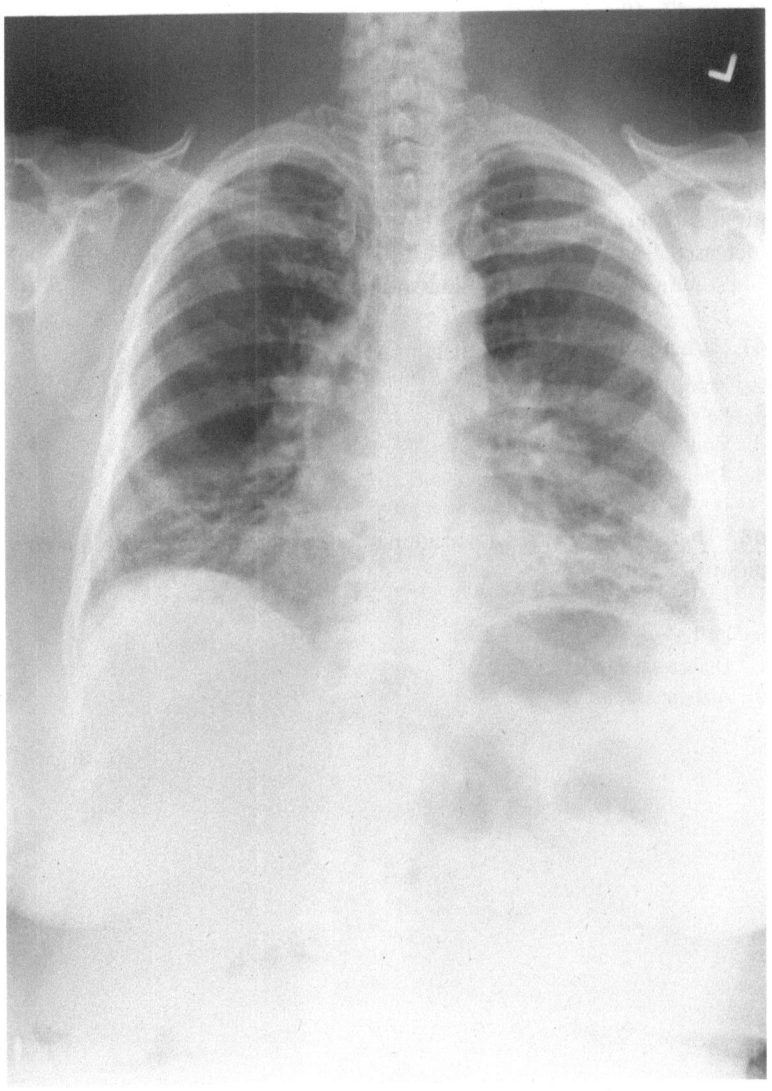

Fig. 25

Items 47–48

A 65-year-old woman from Honduras complains of arthralgias and difficulty getting out of a chair and doing her daily chores at home. She has muscle aches and generalized weakness, dyspnea, and cough. On physical examination, vital signs are: pulse 98 bpm; temperature normal; respirations 23/min and bilateral crackles on lung exam. Neuro exam reveals proximal muscular weakness with no sensory deficit. CPK and aldolase are increased: sedimentation rate is 120 mm/min. PFT: restrictive pattern. Chest radiograph is shown below in Fig. 26.

47. What is the most likely diagnosis?

a. Paraneoplastic syndrome
b. Polymyositis
c. Sjögren syndrome
d. Scleroderma

48. There is an increased association of one of the following with this condition

a. Carcinoma of the pancreas
b. Diabetes mellitus
c. Diabetes insipidus
d. Alzheimer's disease

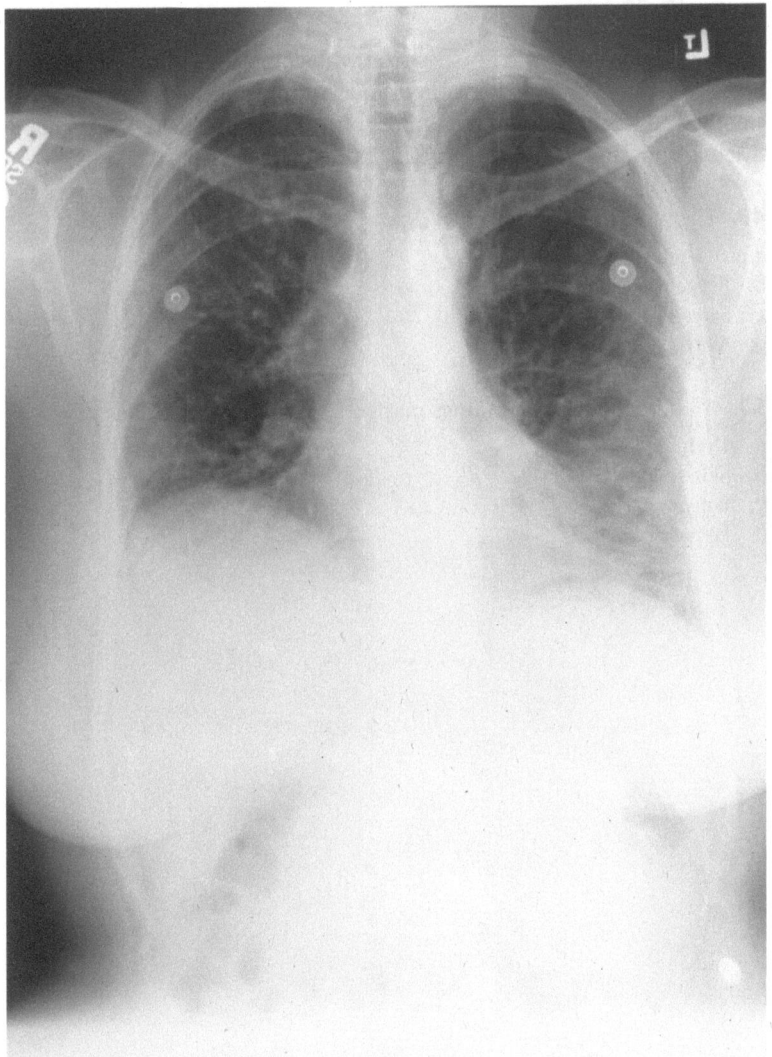

Fig. 26

Items 49–50

A 48-year-old female nurse is seen with complaints of cough. She has been treated for "bronchitis" without much improvement. On exam, she is afebrile and has crackles in the upper zones of the lung field. PPD is negative and sputum for AFB is negative. CXR is shown in Fig. 27.

49. The most likely diagnosis is
a. Tuberculosis
b. Blastomycosis
c. Sarcoidosis
d. Silicosis

50. All of the following findings may be seen in this patient except
a. Uveitis
b. Skin lesion
c. Bony cysts
d. Hypocalcemia

Diffuse Interstitial Disease

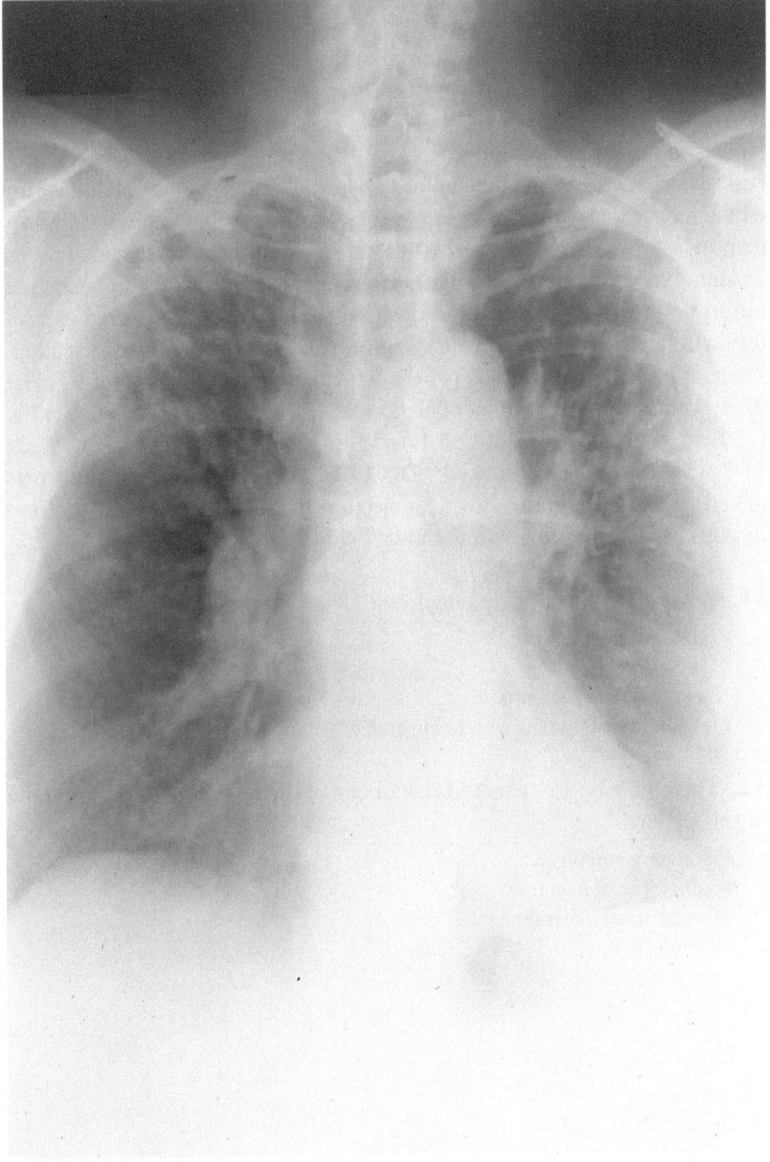

Fig. 27

Items 51–52

A 56-year-old black male nonsmoker is seen with a history of dyspnea on walking two blocks and chronic chest congestion and cough. He has been followed for progressive shortness of breath after his CABG. Recently, he was ill with a flulike illness, but he denies any fever or chills presently. Past history reveals a GI clinic follow-up for inflammatory bowel disease for which he has been on chronic steroid therapy off and on. On physical examination, vital signs are: pulse 110 bpm; temperature normal; respirations 24/min; blood pressure 120/78 mm Hg. General exam: patient appears frail but in no distress. Pertinent findings: coarse rhonchi and scattered expiratory wheeze with squeaks. Heart exam reveals normal S_1-S_2 with no gallop. There is no hepatomegaly or pedal edema. Laboratory data: Hb 11 g; Hct 33%; WBCs 15.0/μL; differential normal. PFTs/spirometry: FVC 3.43 L (78% of predicted); FEV_1: 2.15 L (63% of predicted); FEV_1/FVC% 72%; TLC 5.34 L (69% of predicted); DLCO 14 cc/min/mm Hg (57% of predicted). Echocardiogram shows an ejection fraction of 55% with no focal dyskinesia. Chest radiograph is shown below in Fig. 28.

51. What is the most likely diagnosis?

a. Congestive heart failure
b. COPD
c. Nonspecific pneumonitis
d. Bronchiolitis obliterans with organizing pneumonia (BOOP)

52. There may be an increased risk of one of the following during therapy in this patient

a. Pulmonary embolism
b. Staphylococcal infection
c. Mycobacterial infection
d. HIV infection

Diffuse Interstitial Disease

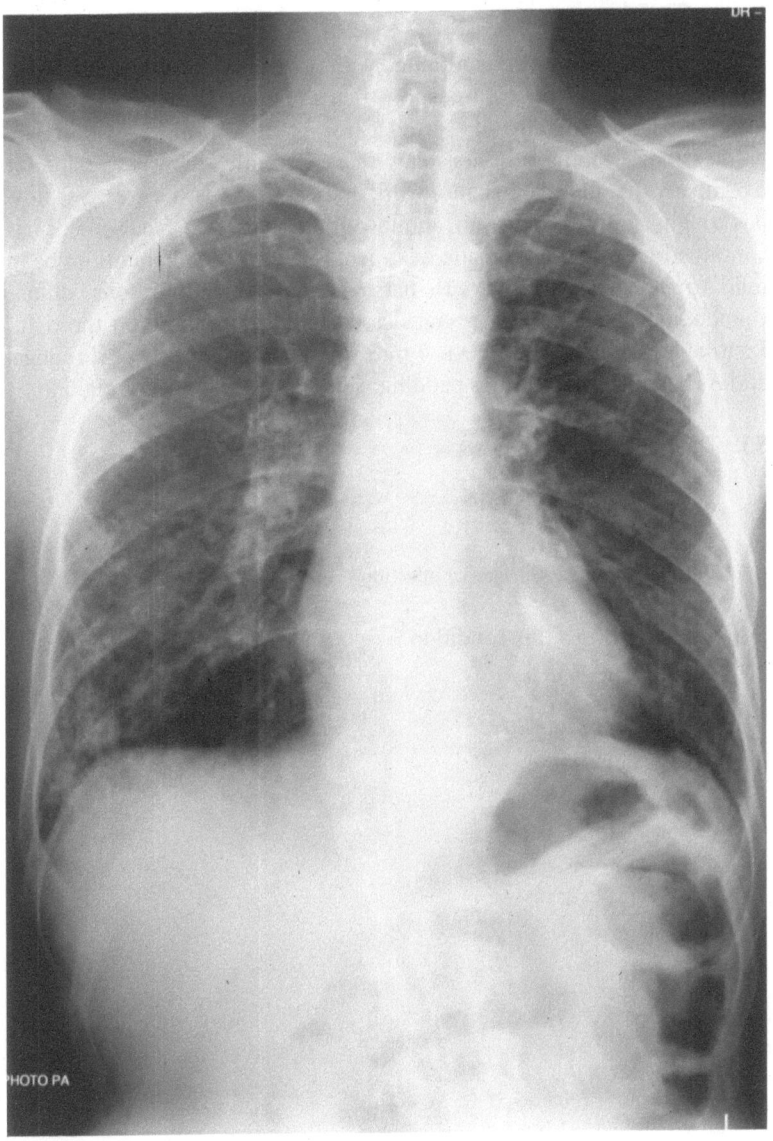

Fig. 28

Items 53–54

A 50-year-old woman is admitted with progressive shortness of breath. She was well until about 2 mo ago, when she noted that she was getting tired and fatigued easily. She gives a history of working as a domestic worker and "cleaning lady" for many years. Recently, she was working for a company that did maintenance work on boats in a marina area. She now has cough, shortness of breath, and low-grade fever with malaise. This has continued despite symptomatic treatment. On exam she is found to be in mild to moderate distress with harsh vesicular breath sounds, diffuse rhonchi, and bilateral basilar crackles on lung exam, more on the right. Routine labs are normal, PPD is 5 mm, and sputum is negative for fungal and AFB smear with cultures pending. Chest x-ray is shown in Fig. 29.

53. The most likely diagnosis is
a. Silicosis
b. Asbestosis
c. Extrinsic allergic alveolitis
d. Nontuberculous mycobacterial infection

54. Associated with this condition is
a. Increased lung volumes
b. Decreased diffusion
c. Peripheral eosinophilia
d. Inorganic dust exposure

Diffuse Interstitial Disease

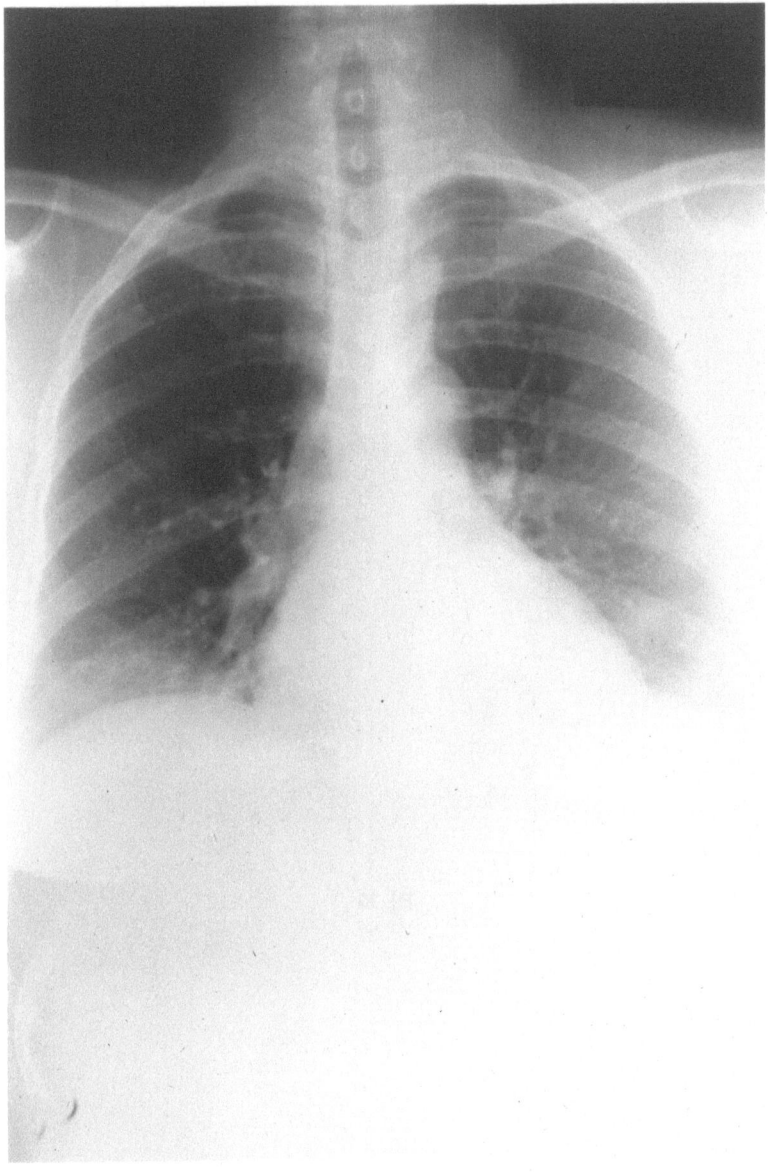

Fig. 29

55. The findings seen on the CXR in Fig. 30 are least likely to be seen in
a. Metastatic adenocarcinoma of the stomach
b. Metastatic carcinoma of the breast
c. Carcinoma of the pancreas
d. Renal cell carcinoma

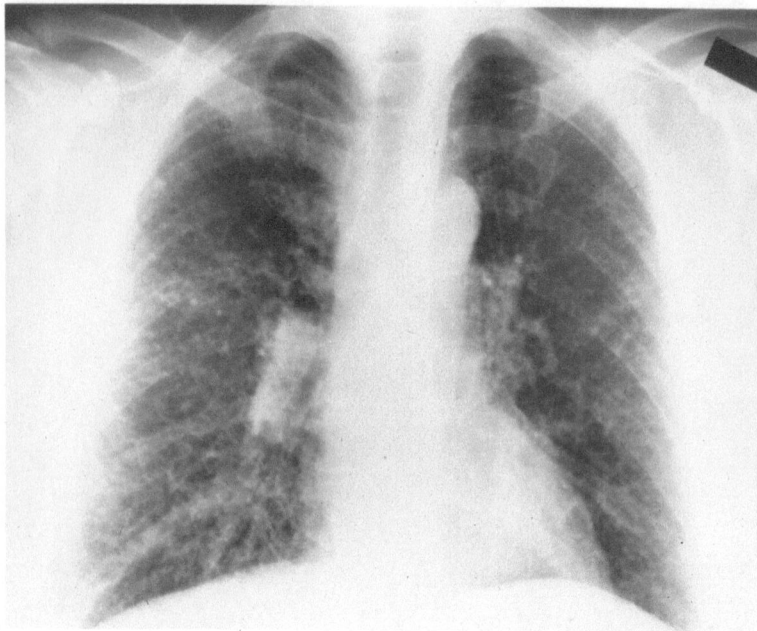

Fig. 30

Diffuse Interstitial Disease

Answers

Description of X-rays in This Chapter

Figure 25. This x-ray shows a bilateral linear reticular and small cystic "honeycombing" pattern in the lower zone. There is hilar prominence without definite vascular or nodal enlargement. The cardiac shadows appear normal. This is consistent with the pattern seen in usual interstitial fibrosis.

Figure 26. This x-ray shows a bilateral interstitial pattern with lower zone predominance. Hilar and cardiac shadows appear normal. The interstitial pattern is more prominent in the left lung. The right diaphragm is raised and the lung volumes appear small.

Figure 27. A bilateral upper zone interstitial pattern is seen with hilar and paratracheal adenopathy. Lung volumes are normal. Cardiac size is normal.

Figure 28. This x-ray shows a bilateral linear-nodular pattern with patchy peripheral distribution. Cardiac size is normal. Cardiophrenic and costophrenic angles appear clear. This is consistent with a nonspecific interstitial pattern.

Figure 29. This x-ray shows normal lung volumes with increased reticular and linear markings in both lower zones, predominantly on the right. The horizontal fissure is displaced downward and there is crowding of the vessels in the right lower lung zone suggesting loss of volume of the right lower lobe. There is a slight uncoiling of the aorta. No mediastinal, paratracheal, or hilar adenopathy is noted.

Figure 30. This x-ray shows a bilateral reticular linear-nodular pattern with peripheral distribution in the lung fields. Some of the nodules are 3 to 5 mm in size. There are Kerley B lines bilaterally from the bases to the upper lung fields. Cardiac shadows are normal and no cephalization of flow is seen.

General Discussion

Diffuse lung disease encompasses a broad array of patterns and etiologies. In general, diffuse disease processes can involve the airspace, the interstitium, or the airways. Diffuse interstitial lung disease is the most common, although airspace and interstitial disease can coexist. Interstitial lung disease involves the supporting structures that surround the airspace, such as the bronchovascular bundles, fissures, and interlobar and intralobar septa. Smooth septal thickening is seen as a result of cellular or fluid infiltration (refer to Chap. 15). Irregular septal thickening without architectural distortion, referred to as the beaded septal sign, may be seen in lymphangitic carcinomatosis, sarcoidosis, and pneumoconiosis. Honeycombing refers to irreversible fibrosis with coarse pattern and associated architectural distortion as a result of end-stage lung disease. Traction on the pulmonary parenchyma produces cystic spaces and traction bronchiectasis.

Most interstitial lung disease results in reduced lung volume with a restrictive pattern on pulmonary function. However, normal or increased volume can be seen in patients with Langerhans granulomatosis/eosinophilic-granuloma, lymphangiomyomatosis, cystic fibrosis, and sarcoidosis. Patients with emphysema may show interstitial involvement with normal or large lung volume.

Distribution can be helpful. Silicosis is involves predominantly the upper lobe; sarcoid may exhibit upper lobe and midlobe involvement, although fibrosis can have lower lobe distribution also. Asbestosis is predominantly seen in the lower lobes on chest x-ray. Idiopathic pulmonary fibrosis of the usual (UIP) variety is a pathologic entity in which there is no regional uniformity of inflammation and fibrosis; therefore this pathology is characterized as temporally dissimilar. Nonspecific interstitial pneumonitis or cellular interstitial pneumonitis shows uniformity of pathology. Nonspecific pneumonitis is seen in connective tissue disorders, collagen vascular diseases, rheumatoid arthritis, and polymyositis, but may be idiopathic. It is common in hypersensitivity pneumonitis and bronchocentric granulomas. It can also occur in drug-induced interstitial reactions. In rheumatoid arthritis, the pulmonary disease does not correlate with the extent or severity of the underlying arthritis. Pulmonary disease is more common in men who

Diffuse Interstitial Disease Answers 101

have rheumatoid arthritis than in women with RA. In 20% of patients, the lung disease may precede the development of arthritis.

Specific Discussion

44–46. The answers are 44-d, 45-a, 46-b. The clinical symptoms of cough and dyspnea in a 49-year-old woman without any specific arthritis or skin lesions, and the presence of clubbing and bilateral Velcro rales, suggest idiopathic pulmonary fibrosis. This disease has a slightly male predominance and usually presents in the sixth decade. Associated findings in this condition include a positive ANA/RA and an increased sedimentation rate. Increased IgE is not seen in idiopathic pulmonary fibrosis. The pulmonary function test in this condition would show a restrictive pattern. The absence of specific arthritis and skin lesions makes rheumatoid lung or sarcoidosis less likely.

47–48. The answers are 47-b, 48-a. Symptoms of arthralgias and difficulty in movement as well as muscular pain and weakness along with an increased CPK and aldolase suggest polymyositis. Interstitial disease is associated with this condition. About 25% of patients may have an occult malignancy; carcinoma of the pancreas is most common. Other complications include respiratory failure and aspiration. The response to steroid therapy is variable.

49–50. The answers are 49-c, 50-d. The physical signs are inconsistent with an infectious process. The CXR shows hilar, paratracheal LN, and parenchymal disease. Sarcoidosis may be associated with uveitis, skin lesions, bony cysts, and hypercalcemia, which is due to abnormal vitamin D metabolism. Sarcoidosis is a systemic disease of unknown etiology characterized pathologically by widespread development of noncaseating epithelioid cell granulomas, which may resolve or convert to fibrous tissue. The disease most commonly affects hilar lymph nodes and lungs, but uveitis and involvement of other organs such as the liver, spleen, skin, bone, and salivary glands are not rare. Lab studies may show anemia, leukopoenia, elevated SED rates, blood eosinophilia, hypercalcemia, hypercalciuria, and elevated levels of serum angiotensin-converting enzymes. Half of the cases are detected incidentally on chest radiograph. Patients with adenopathy alone are usually asymptomatic, although patients with pulmonary involvement may experience weight loss, fatigue, fever, cough, or shortness of breath. Hemoptysis is rare unless it is associated with end-stage sarcoidosis and a superimposed mycetoma. The disease is most common in African Americans, Puerto Ricans, and West Indians. Women are more susceptible than men. Diagnosis is usually confirmed by transbronchial biopsy, which can demonstrate granulomas despite the absence of radiographic evidence of this peribronchial disease. Adenopathy is the most common manifestation. Symmetrical, hilar, and classically right paratracheal involvement is seen. Unilateral hilar adenopathy is seen in less than 5% of cases. Peripheral "eggshell" lymph node calcification is occasionally seen. Pleural effusion is rare.

Radiographic staging of sarcoid is as follows:

Stage 0: normal finding, 10% at presentation, with the primary problem being nonpulmonary
Stage 1: adenopathy without pulmonary disease, 50% at presentation
Stage 2: adenopathy with pulmonary disease, 30% at presentation
Stage 3: pulmonary disease without adenopathy, 10% at presentation
Stage 4: pulmonary fibrosis, usually as a sequel to stage 3, rare at presentation

Stage 1 disease resolves within a few years in most patients, and less than one-third of patients with stage I disease develop lung disease. Adenopathy is usually present when there is pulmonary disease. The lung involvement results from deposition of noncaseating granulomas along the lymphatic lining of the bronchial vascular bundles and interlobular septa. Findings include small, irregular interstitial and subpleural nodules throughout the lungs. Confluent interstitial infiltrates may be asymmetric, and cavitation is rare. The midzone and upper zone are most commonly involved, whereas the lung periphery and the bases are generally spared. Pulmonary involvement usually resolves but does progress to fibrosis in less than 20% of the cases, with architectural distortion, traction, and pleural thickening. The distribution is often patchy, in contrast to the peripheral lower lobe distribution of IPF. Occasionally, pulmonary sarcoidosis may appear as ground-glass opacities, patchy consolidation, or rounded "cannonball" infiltrates described as alveolar sarcoid.

51–52. The answers are 51-d, 52-c. This nonspecific interstitial disease was histologically confirmed as bronchiolitis obliterans with organizing pneumonia (BOOP). There are no signs of CHF. Bronchiolitis refers to inflammation involving the small airways. Proliferative bronchiolitis is a result of organizing intraluminal exudates, and, when associated with inflammation infiltrating the airspace and interstitium, is referred to as BOOP. Typically, it is seen with a history of several weeks of nonproductive cough and dyspnea after an upper respiratory tract infection in a middle-aged person. A prolonged course of steroids is needed to control the symptoms. There is an increased risk of mycobacterial infections in patients on chronic steroid therapy.

53–54. The answers are 53-c, 54-b. Inhalation of organic dusts derived from animal dander, proteins, microbial antigens, water reservoirs, etc., can cause hypersensitivity pneumonitis or extrinsic allergic alveolitis. The symptoms of low-grade fever, shortness of breath with progressive deterioration, and the presence of rhonchi and crackles on physical examination suggest hypersensitivity pneumonitis. The chest radiograph is consistent with this diagnosis. There is no specific occupational exposure to silica or asbestos. The chest x-ray is not suggestive of silicosis. Lung volumes are usually maintained or slightly decreased at a later stage and diffusion capacity is decreased. With the exception of acute episodes, the white blood cell count is not elevated and eosinophilia is not usual. The presence in serum of precipitating antibodies (IgG, IgM) to antigens causing the disease is helpful in diagnosis. Therapy requires avoidance of the causative agent. A trial of corticosteroids may help in relieving symptoms in some cases.

55. The answer is d. Lymphangitic carcinomatosis is seen when tumor metastasizes to the interstitium and lymphatics and spreads along the intralobar septa and connecting tissue. It is seen most commonly secondary to metastatic spread of adenocarcinoma of the lung, breast, pancreas, stomach, and colon. Infiltrates are seen more commonly in the lower zones. Hilar adenopathy or pleural effusion may occur. The radiographic appearance of lymphangitic carcinomatosis is variable. Although bilateral disease is usual, unilateral predominance can be seen in adenocarcinoma of the lung, breast, and stomach. Fifty percent of the patients with lymphangitic carcinomatosis may have normal chest x-rays. A high-resolution CT scan will increase the detection in patients with known malignancy and underlying dyspnea.

DIFFUSE AIRSPACE DISEASE

106 Chest Radiology

DIRECTIONS: For each item below, match the scenario with the appropriate x-ray.

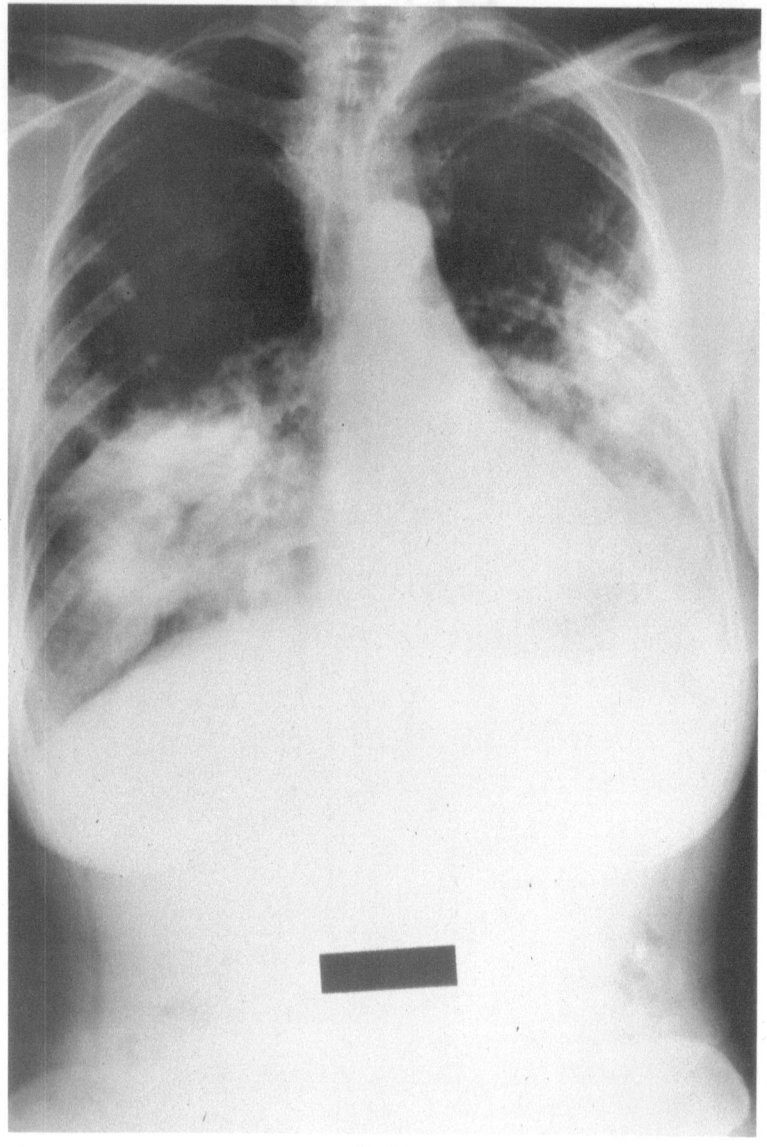

Fig. 31

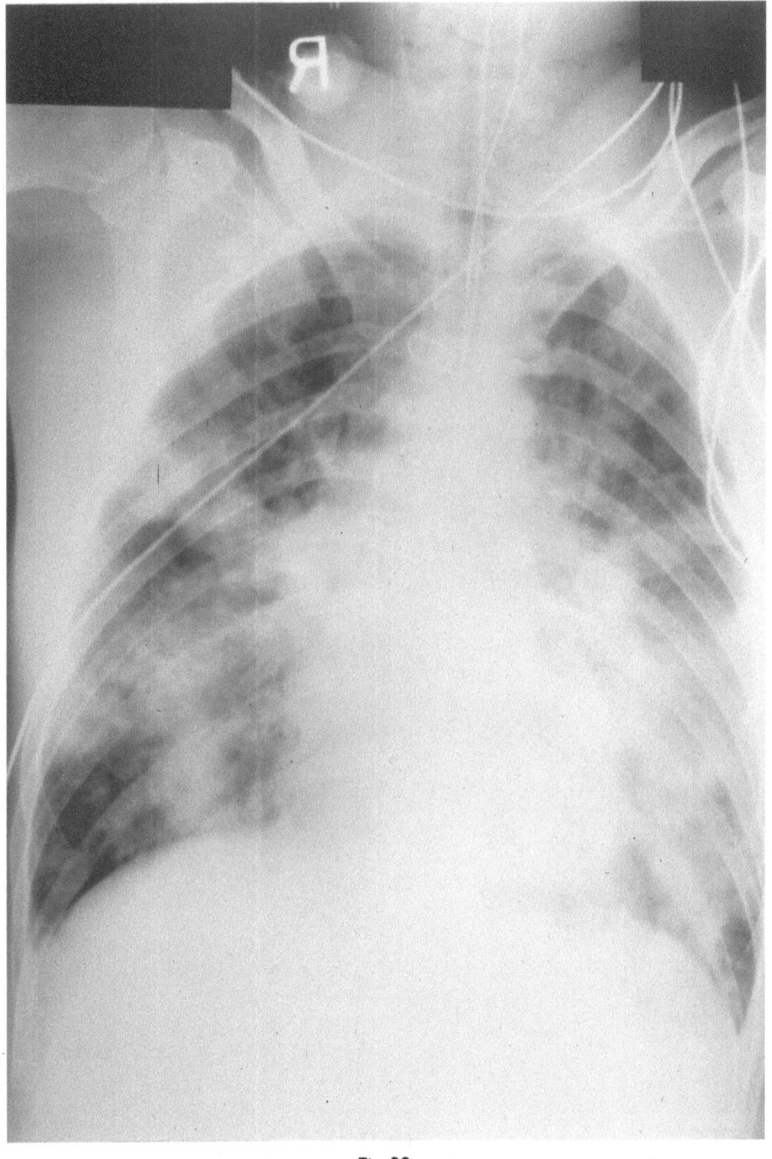

Fig. 32

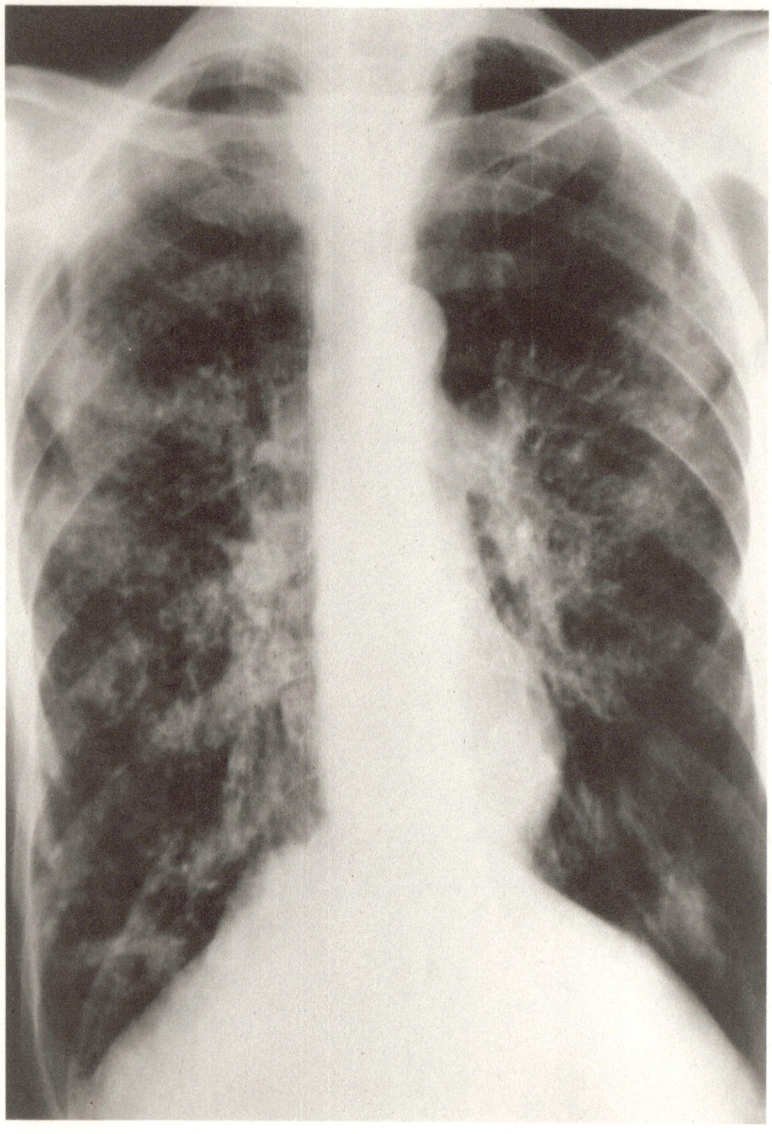

Fig. 33

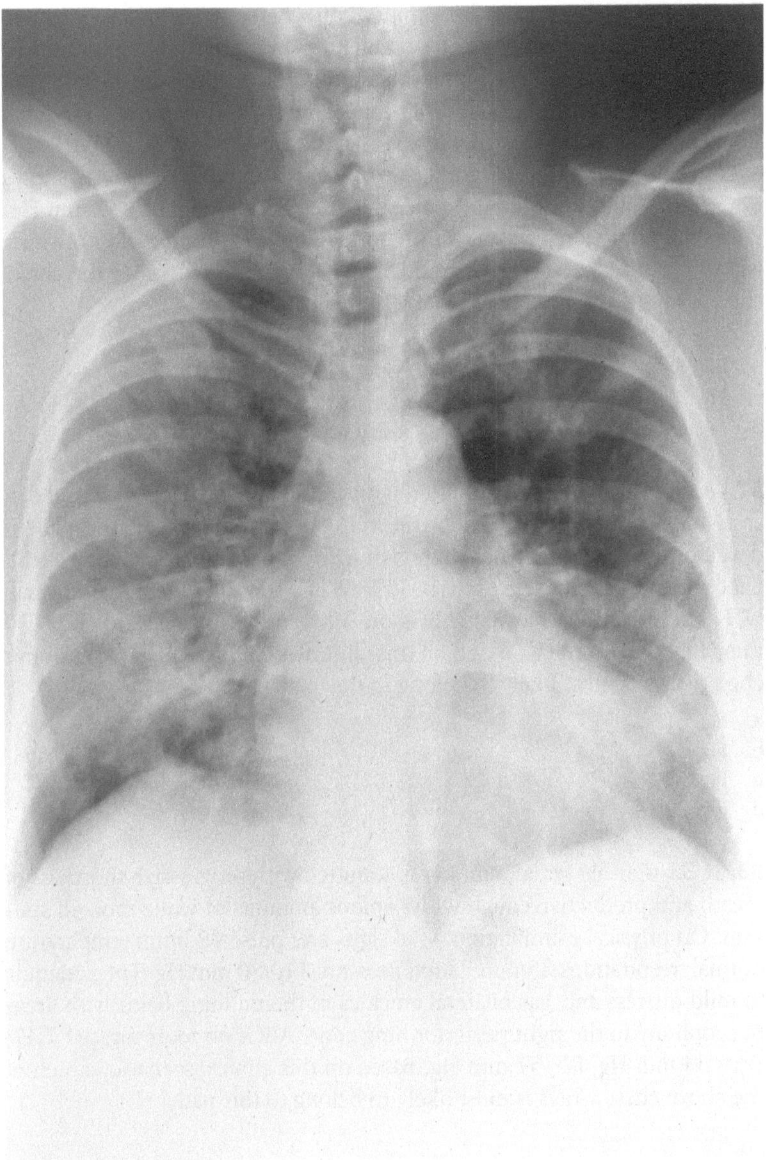

Fig. 34

56. A 44-year-old woman is admitted with hemoptysis and progressive shortness of breath. On physical examination, her vital signs are: pulse 110 bpm; temperature 99°F; respirations 22/min; blood pressure 118/68 mm Hg. She is in mild distress and her lung exam is normal except for occasional crackles. Laboratory data: Hb 9.8 g/dL; Hct 30%; WBCs 9.0/μL; differential normal; BUN 46 g/dL; creatinine 1.9 mg/dL. Urinalysis shows RBC casts. ABGs on room air: pH 7.42; P_{CO_2} 38 mm Hg; P_{O_2} 72 mm Hg. Pulmonary function tests are within normal limits except for DLCO, which is 110% of predicted. Based on this clinical scenario, which of the above chest x-rays is most likely to belong to this patient?

a. Fig. 31
b. Fig. 32
c. Fig. 33
d. Fig. 34

57. A 62-year-old man is admitted with chest pain. He has four-vessel disease and undergoes CABG. On the third postoperative day, the patient develops increasing shortness of breath with diffuse crackles on lung exam. Laboratory data: Hb 12 g/dL; Hct 36%; WBCs 9.8/μL; differential normal; BUN and creatinine normal. ABGs on 3% Ventimask: pH 7.50; P_{CO_2} 30 mm Hg; P_{O_2} 87 mm Hg. Based on this clinical scenario, which of the above chest x-rays is most likely to belong to this patient?

a. Fig. 31
b. Fig. 32
c. Fig. 33
d. Fig. 34

58. A 38-year-old female smoker is admitted with progressive shortness of breath and productive cough with copious amounts of white mucoid sputum. On physical examination, vital signs are: pulse 98 bpm; temperature normal; respirations 35/min; blood pressure 110/80 mm Hg. The patient is in mild distress and has bilateral crackles in the midlung fields with areas of egophony in the right posterior lung zone. ABGs on room air: pH 7.47; P_{CO_2} 34 mm Hg; P_{O_2} 57 mm Hg. Based on this clinical scenario, which of the above chest x-rays is most likely to belong to this patient?

a. Fig. 31
b. Fig. 32
c. Fig. 33
d. Fig. 34

59. A 72-year-old man with a history of COPD and chronic sputum production, on home O_2, with a long-standing history of reflux esophagitis and difficulty swallowing, is admitted with shortness of breath and fever. On physical examination, his vital signs are: pulse 128 bpm; temperature 101°F; respirations 34/min; blood pressure: 98/65 mm Hg. He appears frail and has bilateral crackles and rhonchi on lung exam. Laboratory data: Hb 10 g/dL; Hct 30%; WBCs 15.8/µL; BUN 56 mg/dL; creatinine 2.8 mg/dL; sodium 128 mEq/L; potassium 3.2 mEq/L. ABGs on room air: pH 7.5; P_{CO_2} 34 mm Hg; P_{O_2} 48 mm Hg. Based on this clinical scenario, which of the above chest x-rays is most likely to belong to this patient?
a. Fig. 31
b. Fig. 32
c. Fig. 33
d. Fig. 34

DIFFUSE AIRSPACE DISEASE

Answers

Description of X-rays in This Chapter

Figure 31. This x-ray shows bilateral airspace opacities that are patchy in nature with lower zone segmental/lobar distribution. Air bronchograms are seen within the opacities.

Figure 32. Sternal wires are seen indicating sternotomy s/p CABG. There are diffuse airspace opacities. Cardiac size is at the upper limits of normal; marked increased hilar fullness suggests increased pulmonary vasculature.

Figure 33. This CXR shows increased lung volume with signs of hyperinflation and flattened diaphragm consistent with COPD/emphysema. The cardiac shadow is narrow and tubular in shape. Bilateral patchy opacities are seen throughout the lung fields.

Figure 34. Diffuse bilateral airspace opacities with air bronchograms are seen throughout the lung fields.

General Discussion

Diffuse lung disease encompasses a broad array of patterns and etiologies, often with coexisting airspace and interstitial disease. Causes of diffuse lung opacification involving the airspaces include those associated with the presence of blood, pus, fluid, protein, or cells in the lung parenchymal airspaces. The common etiological diagnoses based on these causes are pulmonary hemorrhagic syndromes, pneumonia, pulmonary edema, alveolar proteinosis, and bronchoalveolar carcinoma. These x-ray changes may overlap and appear similar in all these conditions. With diffuse airspace disease, clinical correlation is very important in suggesting a specific diagnosis.

Specific Discussion

56. The answer is d. The clinical scenario of hemoptysis with shortness of breath and diffuse airspace opacity is consistent with pulmonary hemorrhage. Increased DLCO is consistent with intraalveolar hemorrhage. Causes of diffuse pulmonary hemorrhage include vasculitis/capillaritis with its systemic causes and manifestations, pulmonary-renal syndromes such as Goodpasture syndrome, bleeding diathesis in an immune-compromised host, or idiopathic hemosiderosis.

57. The answer is b. This patient has undergone CABG and has developed pulmonary edema and acute respiratory distress syndrome (ARDS). Sometimes referred to as shock lung, ARDS encompasses a syndrome that refers to a constellation of respiratory distress, marked dyspnea, hypoxemia, and diffused airspace consolidation. It is as a result of medical or traumatic insult causing diffuse alveolar damage. Common causes include septic or hemorrhagic shock, trauma, burns, infection, aspiration, drug intoxication, pneumonia, embolism, near-drowning, inhalational injury, and anaphylaxis. ARDS generally takes a few days to develop, and there may be a delay between the onset of symptoms and the appearance of radiographic signs. There is usually no cardiomegaly or pleural effusion except when associated with CHF. Lung volumes and lung compliance are reduced. Fibrosis may develop, and later complications including pneumothorax, pneumomediastinum, and pneumonia are frequent. Pulmonary edema may result from increased pulmonary venous pressure (hydrostatic pulmonary edema) due to congestive heart failure or volume overload.

58. The answer is a. The clinical syndrome suggests bronchorrhea. This symptom is uncommon and is reported with bronchoalveolar carcinoma (BAC) and bronchiectasis. Occasionally, desquamative interstitial pneumonitis and usual interstitial pneumonitis may produce large amount of mucoid phlegm. Bronchoalveolar carcinoma primarily arises from type 2 pneumocytes in the alveoli or Clara cells from the terminal bronchioles. Although different subsets have been described pathologically, these do not appear to have any prognostic significance. X-ray findings have a better prognostic significance. BAC can present as a localized lesion, as a solitary pulmonary nodule, or as focal consolidation simulating pneumonia. A multinodular or miliary pattern may occur. If BAC is multifocal, it usually has a poor prognosis. Adenopathy, effusion, and cavitation are uncommon. CT patterns may show airspace disease and bulging fissures or a "crazy paving" pattern. Bronchoalveolar carcinoma is classified as a subtype of adenocarcinoma that has a tendency to spread locally through the lung structure and stroma. Bronchoalveolar carcinoma accounts for 9% of all lung tumors and is increasing in prevalence. Other features are a high occurrence in nonsmokers and a comparatively high female-to-male ratio. Survival is usually less than 3 years among patients with diffuse disease. Lobar consolidation is associated with poor prognosis.

59. The answer is c. Aspiration pneumonia can occur in any patient with swallowing difficulty. It frequently presents with a nonspecific diffuse airspace infiltrate on the CXR. Pneumonia usually results from aspiration of infected material from the oral pharynx and esophagus into the respiratory tract. This is usually seen in debilitated or unconscious patients and in individuals with neuromuscular disease or esophageal disease with reflux. The posterior segment of the right upper lobe or the superior segment of the right lower lobe is commonly affected. Bilateral lower lobe basilar infiltrates also suggest aspiration pneumonia. Continuous low-grade aspiration may produce diffuse infiltrates as seen in this patient. Although 90% of the time anaerobic bacteria are found, infection is usually polymicrobial.

Focal Airspace Homogeneous Opacities

DIRECTIONS: Each item below contains a question or incomplete statement followed by suggested responses. Select the **one best** response to each question.

Items 60–62

A 56-year-old male smoker is admitted with shortness of breath, right-sided chest wall pain, and productive cough. He has a past history of seizure disorder and is on anticonvulsants. Dilantin level is within therapeutic range. On examination, there is dullness to percussion in the right upper zone with decreased breath sounds. Sputum for AFB and fungi are negative on initial smear and cultures are pending. CXR is shown in Fig. 35.

60. The most likely diagnosis is

a. Bronchogenic cancer
b. Aspiration pneumonia
c. Fungal pneumonia
d. TB

61. The next step in the management of this patient should be

a. Start anti-TB medications till cultures are final
b. Start Rx with itraconazole
c. Place patient on antireflux and aspiration precautions
d. Consult for bronchoscopy

62. The associated finding that would be least likely in this patient is

a. Gingival hyperplasia
b. Lateral nystagmus
c. Hypercalcemia
d. Erythema nodosum

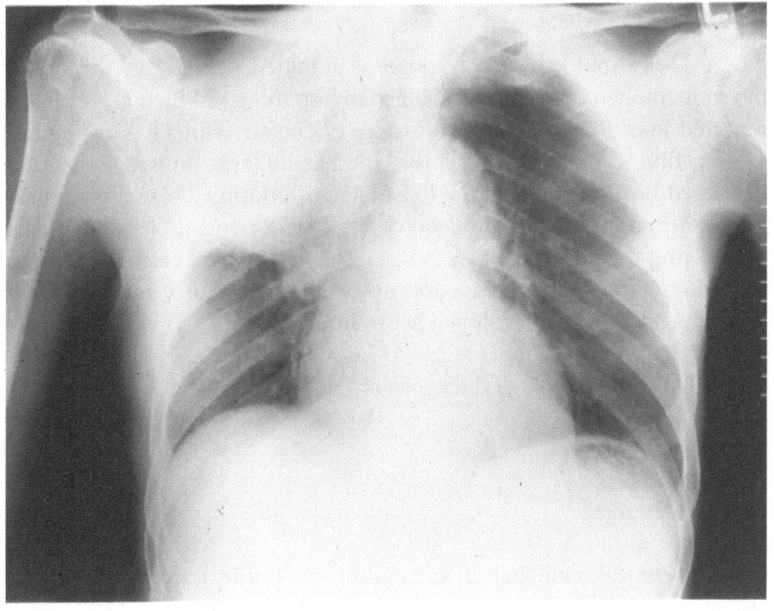

Fig. 35

Items 63–64

A 32-year-old female nonsmoker is admitted with a 5-wk history of intermittent hemoptysis. She denies any sputum production, fever, or repeated infections. There is no history of contact with TB. On physical examination, the patient is afebrile; she has dullness on percussion and decreased breath sounds in the LLL zone posteriorly. CV exam is normal. PPD is 4-mm induration. Bronchoscopy shows a polypoid lesion partially obstructing the left lower lobe orifice. This lesion bled easily during the procedure. Bronchial washings are negative for malignancy and the biopsy is pending. Chest x-ray is shown below in Fig. 36.

63. What is the radiological diagnosis?

a. LLL pneumonia
b. LLL atelectasis
c. Pneumothorax
d. Pleural effusion

64. The clinical, radiological, and endoscopic features described are consistent with

a. Endobronchial carcinoid
b. Bronchiectasis
c. Bronchoalveolar cell carcinoma
d. Primary TB

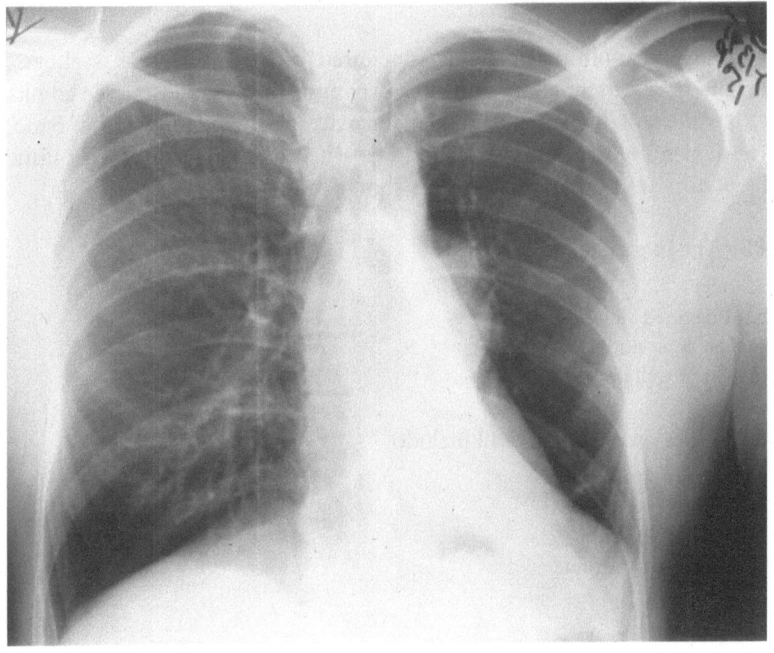

Fig. 36

Items 65–66

A 56-year-old male smoker is referred with symptoms of weakness, dizziness, and right chest pain after playing with his grandson. He admits to having pain in the right shoulder and axilla off and on for the prior 6 mo. He denies any exposure to TB and has a negative PPD skin test. Routine laboratory tests are normal. CXR is shown in Fig. 37.

65. The most likely diagnosis is
a. TB
b. Fractured clavicle
c. Pancoast tumor
d. Chest wall lipoma

66. Associated findings will include
a. Horner syndrome
b. Lofgren syndrome
c. Sjögren syndrome
d. Hertford syndrome

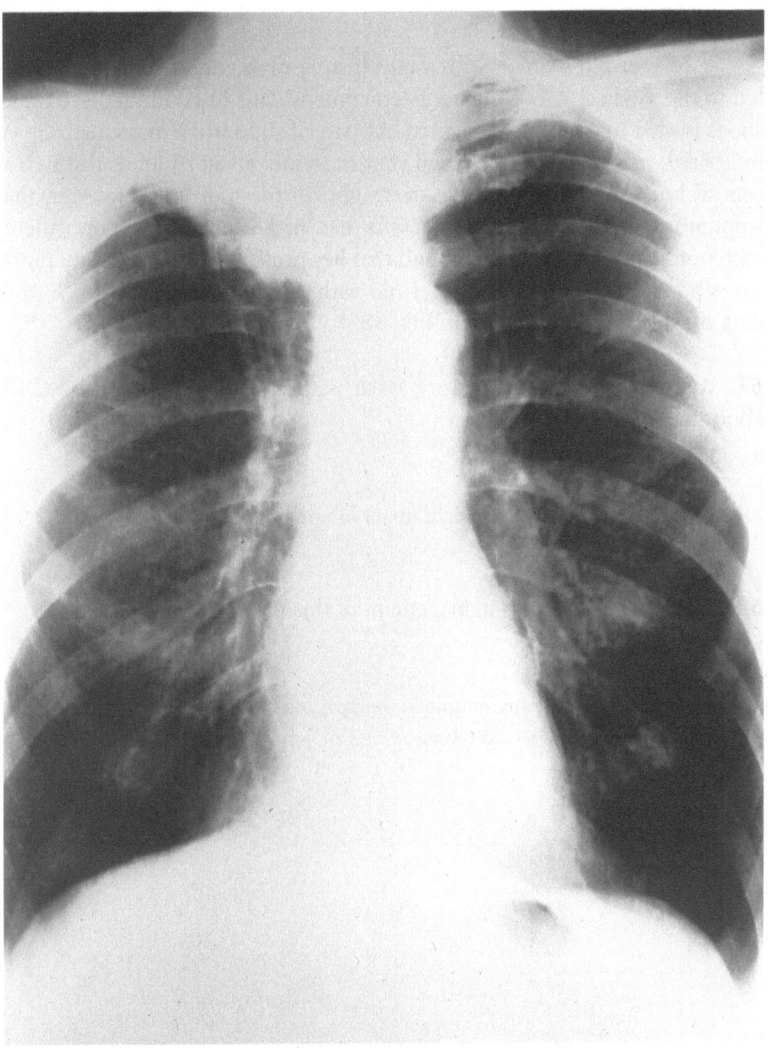

Fig. 37

Items 67–68

A 26-year-old woman with a past history of seizure disorder is admitted to the medical ICU with status epilepticus. Due to continued seizures, she is placed in a barbiturate coma. As part of supportive measures, she is intubated, placed on a mechanical ventilator, and given IV fluids through a central line. She remains stable overnight. In the morning, however, the respiratory therapist reports that she has had excessive mucopurulent secretions throughout the night and that her peak and plateau airway pressures have risen 20 cm. She is febrile with a temperature of 100.2°F the next morning. CXR is shown in Fig. 38.

67. Based on the clinical history, what is the likely etiology of the CXR abnormality?
a. Right-sided hemothorax
b. Lung abscess
c. Aspiration pneumonia with right upper lobe atelectasis
d. Lung contusion

68. An important step in management of this patient would be
a. Chest tube placement
b. Thoracotomy
c. Fiberoptic bronchoscopy, antibiotic therapy, and chest physiotherapy
d. Abrupt cessation of barbiturates

Focal Airspace Homogeneous Opacities 123

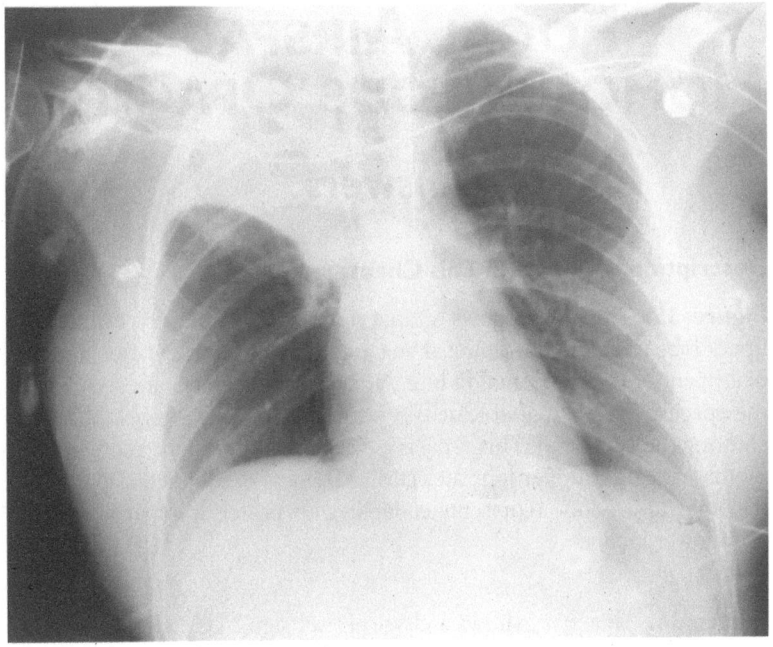

Fig. 38

FOCAL AIRSPACE HOMOGENEOUS OPACITIES

Answers

Description of X-rays in This Chapter

Figure 35. This x-ray shows a large homogeneous density in the right upper lobe with loss of volume as suggested by tracheal deviation and displacement of the horizontal fissure. No air bronchograms are seen within the opacity. There is a double density within the opacity, suggesting a mass abutting the chest wall. This x-ray is consistent with postobstructive pneumonia with right upper lobe atelectasis. The less dense medial portion of the right upper lobe represents collapse with posterior expansion of the right lower lobe.

Figure 36. This x-ray shows a classical "sail sign," i.e., a double density seen in the retrocardiac area. This opacity has a homogeneous pattern with no air bronchograms. The left cardiac silhouette is clear. This is left lower lobe collapse/atelectasis.

Figure 37. This x-ray shows a right upper lobe homogeneous opacity merging with the right paratracheal area in the apical segment. This is consistent with a Pancoast tumor. The right clavicle is obscured in its medial aspect but does not show any fracture or erosion. Underlying hyperinflation is seen in all lung fields. The intercostal spaces in the right upper lobe region are diminished. The soft tissue shadows are similar bilaterally above the clavicles.

Figure 38. This x-ray shows homogeneous opacity in the right upper lobe with a marked shift of the horizontal fissure. No air bronchograms are seen. This is consistent with right upper lobe atelectasis. There is a small bump near the hilum in the curve of the minor fissure that may represent a proximal mass.

General Discussion

Pulmonary collapse and *atelectasis* are terms used interchangeably. Associated with atelectasis or "airlessness" of a segment or lobe is homogeneous increased density and usually loss of volume in that lobe. The x-ray signs of lobar atelectasis may be divided into direct and indirect signs. The direct sign is the displacement of the fissure. The indirect signs are local increase in density, elevation of the hemidiaphragm, displacement of the mediastinum, compensatory hyperinflation and displacement of the hilum, approximation of the ribs, absence of air bronchogram, and absence of visibility of the interlobar artery. This sign is especially seen in left lower lobe atelectasis. Most left lower lobe collapse involves the basilar segments. The direction of the collapse is inferior, medial, or posterior and forms a triangle density seen in the medial posterior/inferior portion of the chest. The ipsilateral hilum is pulled inferiorly and decreases in size.

Pulmonary atelectasis or collapse on chest radiograph has been well described. The terms *atelectasis* and *collapse* have been used interchangeably and at times confusingly. One of the most reliable signs of pulmonary collapse and loss of volume is the displacement of the fissures and mediastinal structures. Several types of atelectasis have been described based upon the etiology. *Obstructive* atelectasis is the most common form and is the result of endobronchial tumors, foreign bodies, or mucus plugging. *Compressive* atelectasis is the result of adjacent masses that compress the normal lung. *Passive* atelectasis occurs as a result of pleural effusion compressing the lung and leaving insufficient space for the lung to expand on inspiration. *Adhesive* atelectasis is commonly seen in newborns and is associated with hyaline membrane disease. When seen in adults, it is associated with pulmonary embolism. *Cicatrizing* atelectasis is a result of pulmonary fibrosis after organizing pneumonia or radiation therapy. *Rounded* atelectasis is thought to represent a sequela of previous pleural adhesion. Asbestos pleural effusion is the usual cause of rounded atelectasis; it is seen radiographically in the dorsal portion of the lung base. A swirling of the pulmonary vessels and bronchi produces a cometlike tail on the medial aspect of the atelectatic lung, with thickening of the adjacent pleura.

Specific Discussion

60–62. The answers are 60-a, 61-d, 62-d. The clinical signs of atelectasis as well as absence of any symptoms of pneumonia suggest bronchogenic carcinoma with right upper lobe atelectasis. Other choices present as non-homogeneous airspace disease with either air bronchograms or cavity formation. Bronchoscopy would confirm whether an endobronchial carcinoma is causing this atelectasis. Associated findings in this clinical history would include signs of Dilantin use such as gingival hyperplasia and lateral nystagmus. Bronchogenic carcinoma may be associated with hypercalcemia. Erythema nodosum is not seen in bronchogenic carcinoma and is usually associated with sarcoidosis or fungal disease.

63–64. The answers are 63-b, 64-a. The presence of a polypoid lesion obstructing the left lower lobe orifice is the cause of the left lower lobe atelectasis seen on the x-ray. The absence of air bronchograms is evidence against pneumonia, and failure to see the visceral pleural line with a collapsed lung rules out pneumothorax. There is no evidence of pleural disease and no pleural effusion is seen. The clinical and radiological features are consistent with endobronchial carcinoid. The absence of cystic or multicystic opacities and the lack of sputum rule out bronchiectasis and alveolar cell carcinoma. Primary TB usually presents as pneumonia and is inconsistent with the x-ray shown.

65–66. The answers are 65-c, 66-a. The homogeneous opacity in the apical region is consistent with superior sulcus tumor (Pancoast tumor). This tumor invades the brachial plexus locally and is often associated with pain in the ulnar nerve distribution. It is also associated with Horner syndrome, i.e., anhydrosis, myosis, and ptosis. Lofgren syndrome is associated with sarcoidosis and is a triad of polyarticular arthritis, erythema nodosum, and bilateral hilar adenopathy. Sjögren syndrome may be primary or secondary to another connective tissue disorder and is also known as the sicca syndrome (due to its attendant triad of xerostomia, dry eyes, and arthritis). Hertford syndrome is a uveoparotid fever associated with sarcoidosis. The chest x-ray finding is inconsistent with any of the latter conditions mentioned.

67–68. The answers are 67-c, 68-c. The clinical history as well as the homogeneous density seen in the right upper lobe are consistent with right upper lobe atelectasis. Complications of central line placement may include lung contusion or hemothorax, but the x-ray findings usually show an expanding density. The clinical history with seizure disorder, the subsequent intubation, and the excessive secretions suggest that a mucus plug is probably causing right upper lobe atelectasis. In view of this, the next step in immediate management would be to begin aggressive chest physical therapy, or a bronchoscopy could help dislodge the mucus plug and clear the right upper lobe bronchus.

Focal Airspace Nonhomogeneous Opacities

DIRECTIONS: Each item below contains a question or incomplete statement followed by suggested responses. Select the **one best** response to each question.

Items 69–71

A 41-year-old man from Mississippi presents with a 2-day history of productive cough with yellow sputum and shortness of breath. He has right-sided chest pain that is worse with deep inspiration and complained of fever and chills on the day of admission. On physical exam, he has a temperature of 103°F; pulse 120 bpm; respirations 32/min; BP 128/78. Lung exam reveals increased tactile vocal fremitus on the right side with bronchial breath sounds and egophony in the right upper chest. Laboratory data: WBCs 19,000/μL with 20% bands. PPD is 7 mm and sputum for AFB smear is negative. CXR is shown in Fig. 39.

69. What is the most likely diagnosis?
a. Acute histoplasmosis
b. Community-acquired pneumonia
c. Smear-negative tuberculosis
d. Bronchoalveolar cell carcinoma

70. What is the next step in the management of this patient?
a. Begin empirical trial of anti-TB drugs till culture for TB is back
b. Perform a bronchoscopy
c. Obtain blood cultures and treat as pneumonia
d. Start antifungal therapy

71. Regarding the above diagnosis, which statement is least likely?
a. Seen in non-immune-compromised patients.
b. Prompt improvement usually occurs with treatment.
c. History of malaise and foul-smelling sputum is common.
d. Complications may include pleural effusion.

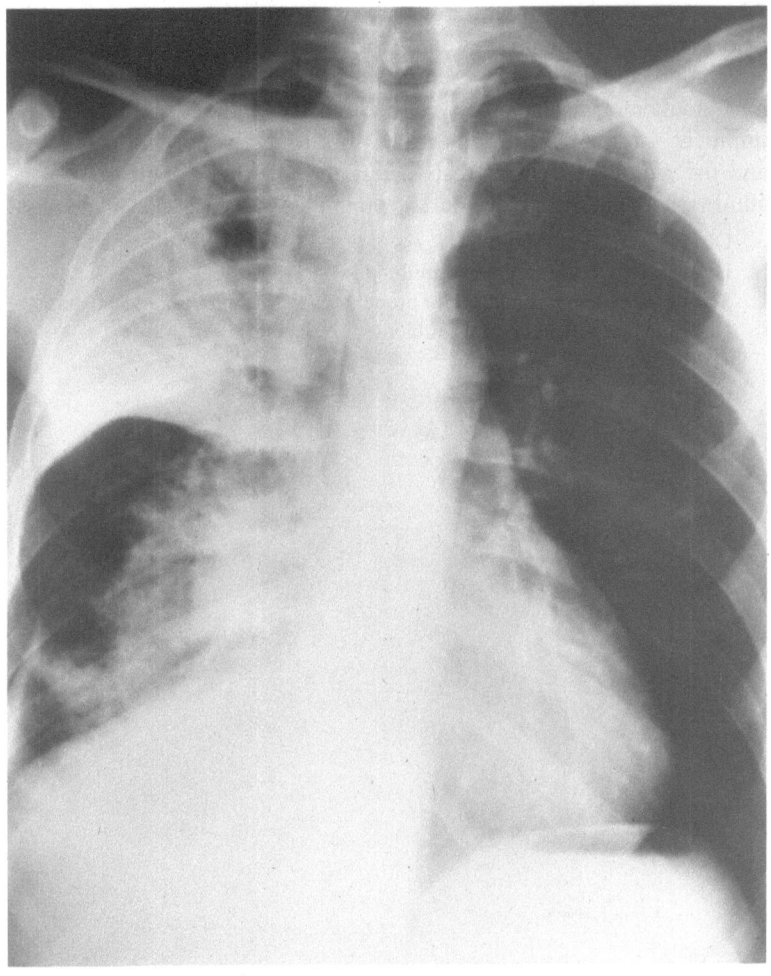

Fig. 39

72. A 69-year-old man with a history of chronic obstructive pulmonary disease/chronic bronchitis is admitted with increasing sputum production, fever, chills, and decreased O_2 saturation. His chest x-ray shows a left lower lobe nonhomogeneous opacity. He is treated with IV antibiotics and improves. On the fourth hospital day, prior to discharge, CXR is repeated and the radiologist reports that there is no change as compared to the admission x-ray. Chest x-rays are shown in Fig. 40. What will you do next?
a. Obtain a CT scan to rule out abscess
b. Defer discharge and resume IV antibiotics
c. Schedule a pulmonary consult for bronchoscopy to improve bronchial drainage
d. Discharge the patient on oral antibiotics

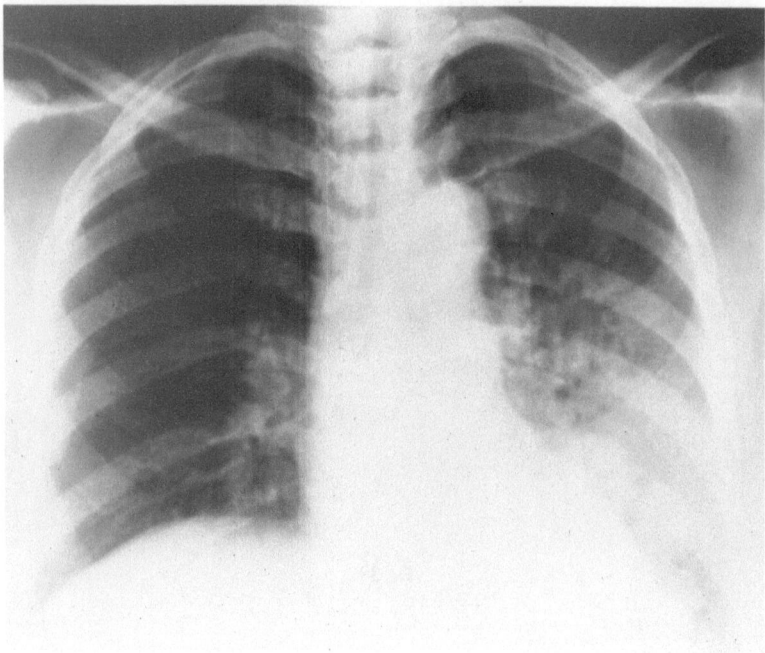

Fig. 40a

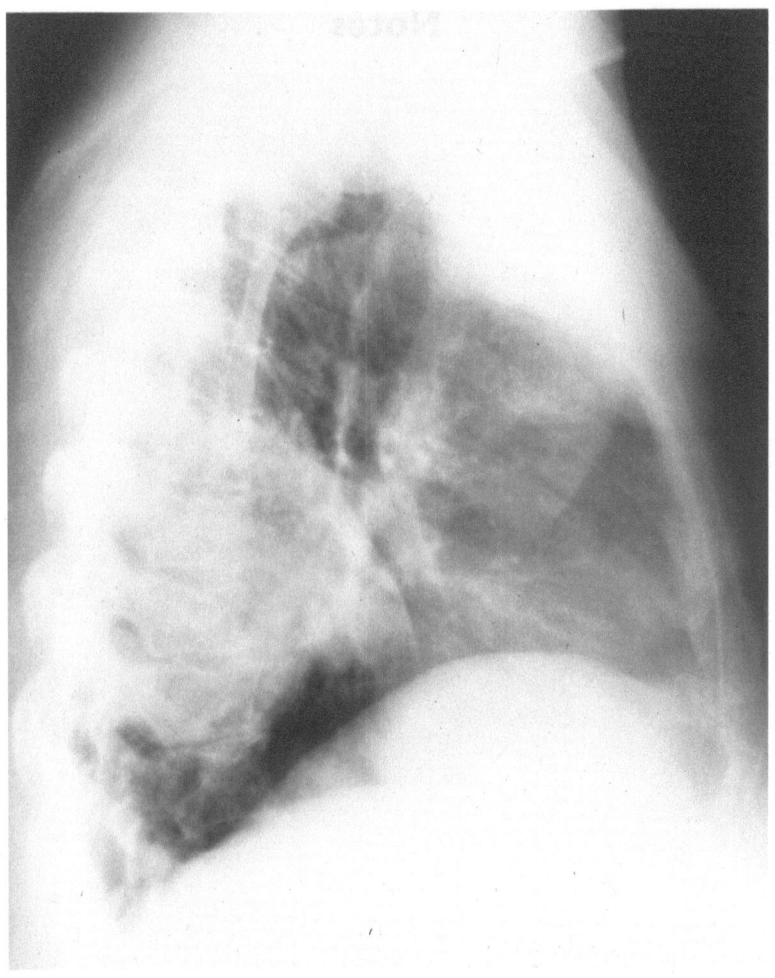

Fig. 40b

Notes

Items 73–75

A 34-year-old woman is admitted with a history of fever, chills, and greenish sputum for 10 days. She has history of ETOH and substance abuse. On physical examination, vital signs are: pulse 113 bpm; temperature 101°F; respirations 25/min; blood pressure 110/78 mm Hg. She looks ill and has crackles with egophony and E to A changes in the right upper lung field. Laboratory data: Hb 12 g/dL; Hct 37%; WBCs 15.0/µL; differential BUN 48 mg/dL; creatinine 1.7 mg/dL. Chest radiographs are shown below in Fig. 41.

73. What is the most likely diagnosis?

a. Klebsiella pneumonia
b. Loculated empyema
c. Postobstructive pneumonia
d. Tuberculosis

74. What is the next management option?

a. Needle aspiration
b. Antibiotics
c. Bronchoscopy
d. CT scan

75. Complications of this condition include all except

a. ARDS
b. Septic shock
c. Hyponatremia
d. Pancreatitis

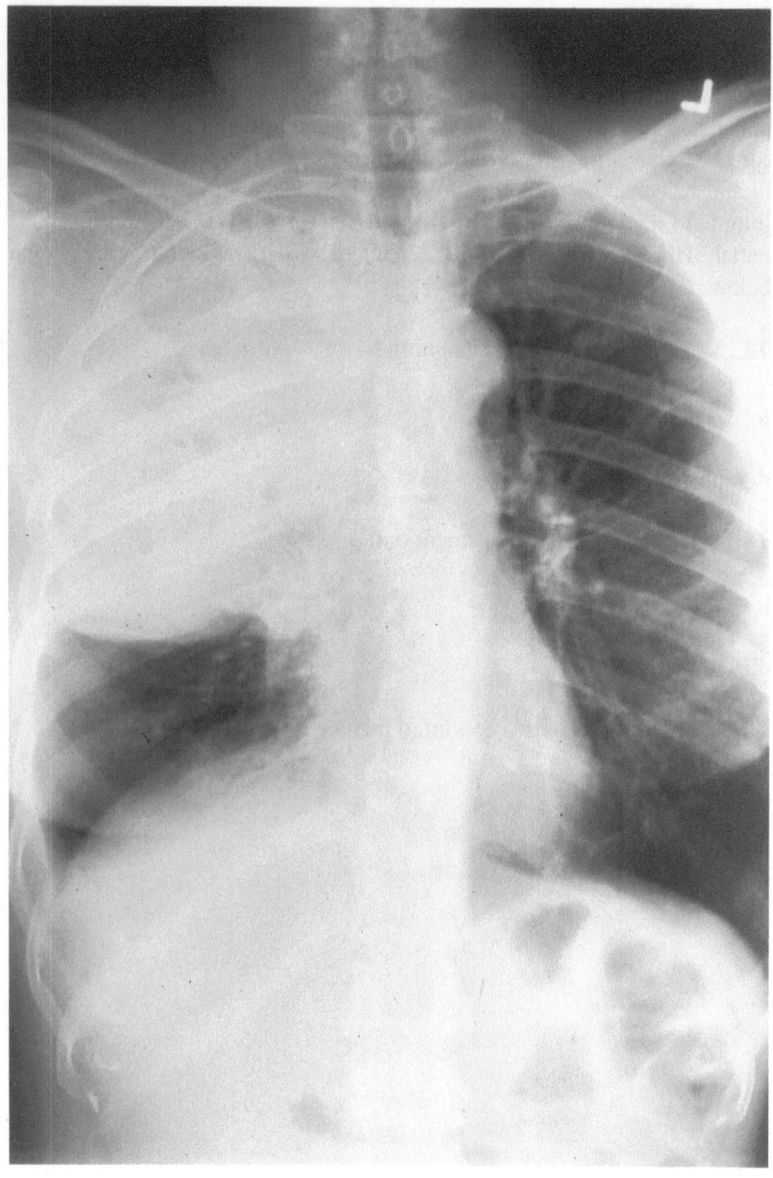

Fig. 41a

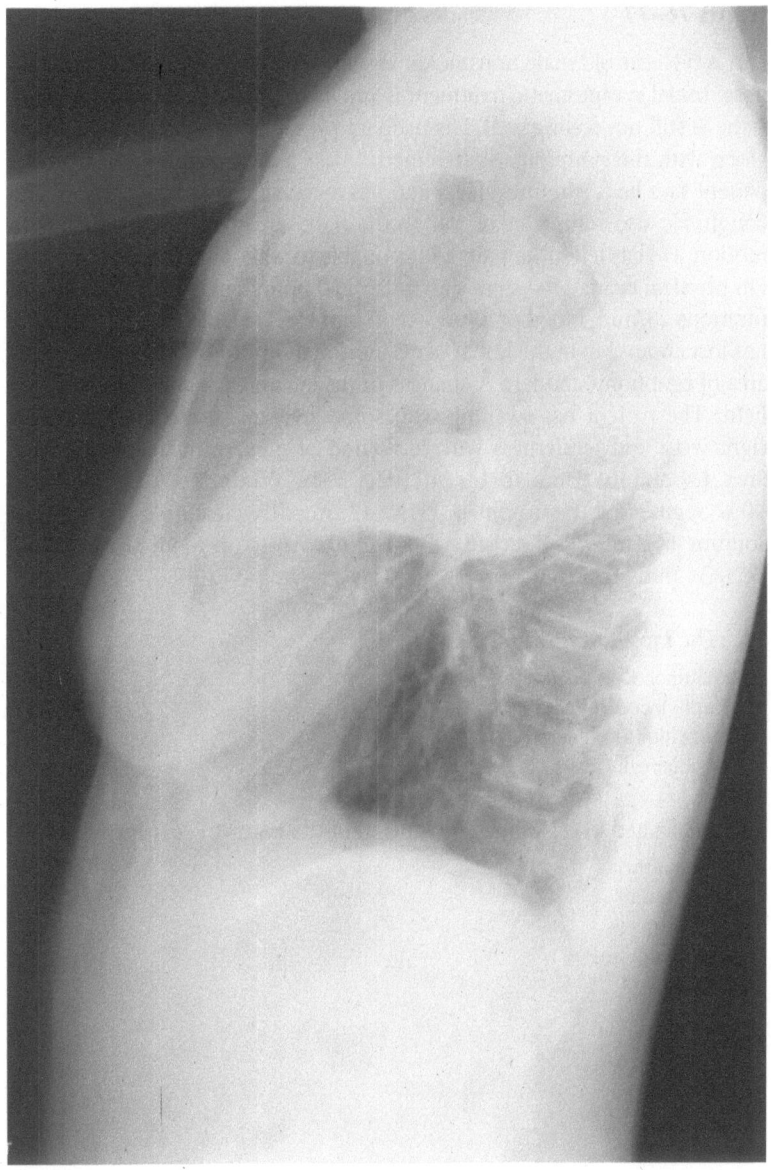

Fig. 41b

Items 76–77

A 54-year-old male nonsmoker is seen with complaints of a flulike illness. Initial symptomatic treatment is provided. Two days later, he returns, as he is still not feeling well. His primary physician prescribes a macrolide along with the symptomatic treatment. After 5 days of this treatment, the patient says he is running a fever and has increasing fatigue, weakness, and cough. He also complains of pain in the right wrist with some difficulty in motion. He has left groin pain and is unable to walk more than a few steps. On physical exam, vital signs are: pulse 110 bpm; temperature 102°F; respirations 24/min; blood pressure 10/68 mm Hg. He looks weak and says he has lost about 8 lb in the last 10 days. Pertinent findings: lung exam reveals area of egophony, and E to A changes in the left anterior and posterior lung field. The patient has swelling with some areas of skin sloughing in the right wrist and tenderness with limitation of movement in the left groin area. Laboratory data: Hb 11 g/dL; Hct 33%; WBCs 16.0/μL; differential 90% segmented neutrophils; BUN 42 mg/dL; creatinine 1.1 mg/dL; sodium 142 mEq/L; potassium 3.4 mEq/L. ABGs on room air: pH 7.45, P_{CO_2} 34 mm Hg; P_{O_2} 65 mm Hg. CXR is shown in Fig. 42.

76. The most likely diagnosis is
a. Pneumococcal pneumonia
b. Staphylococcal Pneumonia
c. Bronchiolitis obliterans
d. Alveolar cell CA

77. Associated findings may include all of the following except
a. Septic arthritis
b. Endocarditis
c. Brain abscess
d. Reye syndrome

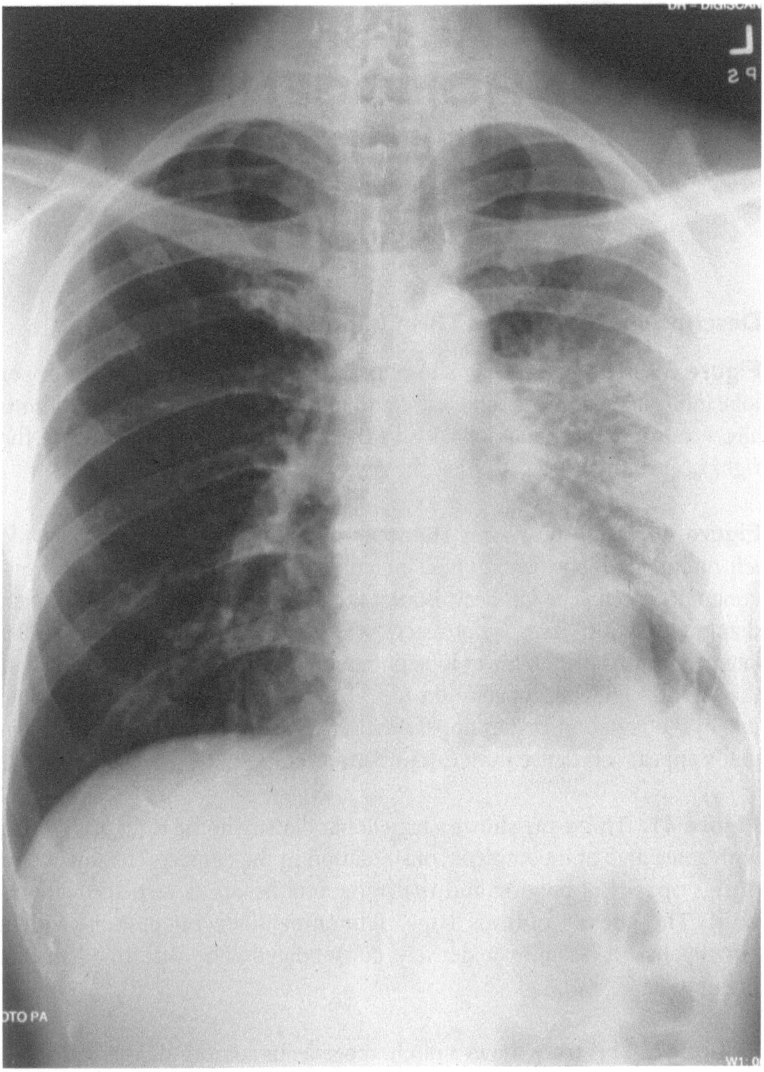

Focal Airspace Nonhomogeneous Opacities

Fig. 42

Focal Airspace Nonhomogeneous Opacities

Answers

Descriptions of X-rays in This Chapter

Figure 39. This chest x-ray shows multilobar opacities. The right upper lobe infiltrate has air bronchograms and minimal loss of volume. Additionally, a non-homogeneous opacity in the right lower zone obscuring the right heart border indicates that the right middle lobe is involved.

Figure 40. This chest x-ray shows an ill-defined, patchy opacity in the left middle and left lower zones. Incomplete consolidation with air bronchogram is seen. The left heart border is clear, but the silhouette of the left diaphragm is lost. This is consistent with the left lower pneumonia. The lateral confirms the left lower lobe pneumonia with opacity posteriorly and the "spine sign," i.e., opacity on top of the normal shadow of the spine makes the vertebral bodies appear denser caudally. (Spinal vertebrae normally appear less dense from top to bottom.)

Figure 41. This x-ray shows a large lobar density in the right upper lobe with some area of incomplete consolidation in the density. The lower end of this opacity is bulging and the horizontal fissure is displaced downward. The lateral confirms large right upper lobe pneumonia with a bulging fissure seen in a densely consolidated lobe due to klebsiella pneumonia.

Figure 42. This x-ray shows a nonhomogeneous airspace density in the left middle and lower zones with areas of incomplete consolidation and evolving pneumatocele formation. The left diaphragm is raised and the trachea appears shifted to the left, suggesting loss of volume of the left lung. There is minimal blunting of the left costophrenic angle, suggesting a left pleural effusion. This CXR is consistent with the left lower lobe necrotizing pneumonia with loss of volume, which can be seen in staphylococcal pneumonia.

General Discussion

The classical radiological signs of pneumonia include a nonhomogenous opacity that has air bronchograms and that may have segmental or lobar distribution. Various "silhouette signs" (i.e., loss of diaphragm margin for lower lobes and loss of heart border for anteriorly placed middle lobe or lingula) are used to determine which lobes are involved. The "spine sign" on a lateral film indicates lower lobe involvement and is especially useful in determining the involvement of the superior segment of the lower lobe. Signs of cavities or breakdown suggest necrotizing gram-negative/mixed/anaerobic infection. Pneumonia occasionally may present as a round density. A nonresolving infiltrate after 4 to 6 wk usually suggests underlying pathology such as an endobronchial lesion.

In approximately 50% of patients with community-acquired pneumonia (CAP), an etiologic diagnosis cannot be made. The common known causes of CAP are bacteria, viruses, and atypical pathogens. The ATS guidelines recommend treatment of patients based on severity of disease and comorbid conditions. *Streptococcus pneumoniae* is the most likely pathogen for all groups, and treatment must include coverage for that organism in all patients. In elderly and chronically ill patients, those with COPD, and even smokers without COPD, coverage must include gram-negative bacteria. Aspiration pneumonia should be considered in those with impaired consciousness or altered swallowing reflexes. About 5% of patients with CAP have *Pseudomonas aeruginosa* identified in their respiratory tract. In the United States, 5% to 35% of pneumococci are now penicillin resistant. Most are intermediate-level resistant and are seen more in immune-compromised and/or chronically ill patients, especially if these patients have received a β-lactam antibiotic in the preceding 3 mo. Mortality rates in severe community-acquired pneumococcal pneumonia exceed 15% but are related to patient host factors and not bacterial resistance. Legionella remains an underestimated and often unidentified pathogen with a high mortality.

Staphylococcal pneumonia is frequently seen in older or debilitated patients, not infrequently occurring as a complication of influenza. The disease is commonly bilateral, starting as patchy multilobar infiltrates. Volume loss in the affected segment with concomitant effusion, pneumatocele, and abscess formation can be seen.

Specific Discussion

69–71. The answers are 69-b, 70-c, 71-c. The acute onset of illness along with the physical examination consistent with pneumonia suggests this to be a community-acquired pneumonia in a healthy host. Although this patient is from an endemic area where histoplasmosis is prevalent, this is not the usual clinical presentation of fungal disease. *S. pneumoniae* is the likely pathogen. The next management step should be to treat the patient after obtaining blood cultures. About 10% of patients with community-acquired pneumococcal pneumonia will have positive blood cultures. This pneumonia usually responds well to treatment. Foul-smelling sputum and a generalized history of chronic malaise are uncommon in community-acquired pneumonia.

72. The answer is d. This patient with chronic obstructive pulmonary disease has left lower lobe pneumonia. The clinical history suggests that the patient improved on the fourth hospital day of treatment. Chest x-ray improvement usually lags behind and does not temporally correspond with clinical change. In this case the patient is improving and therefore the best option is to discharge the patient on continued antibiotics. There is no indication for either deferring the discharge or resuming IV antibiotics on the basis of a nonresolving x-ray at this stage. Bronchoscopy for drainage would not be indicated, and obtaining a CT scan would not alter the treatment or management plan at this stage.

73–75. The answers are 73-a, 74-b, 75-d. The chest x-ray and the clinical picture are consistent with pneumonia. The bulging fissure with a densely consolidated lobe has been described with klebsiella pneumonia, although it can occur more frequently with *S. pneumomiae*. Tuberculosis pneumonia would show cavitary disease with loss of volume. A loculated empyema presents as a pleural base opacity. Based on the diagnosis of pneumonia, the next management step is to start the antibiotics. Because of the immune-compromised status of the patient as well as the extent of the pneumonia, complications would include ARDS and septic shock. Hyponatremia is seen with pneumonia and indicates inappropriate ADH secretion. Although patients with ETOH abuse may have pancreatitis per se, this is not a complication of pneumonia.

76–77. The answers are 76-b, 77-d. The prodrome of a flulike illness and the development of pneumonia along with multisystem involvement suggest a bacteremic process. Both staphylococcal and pneumococcal pneumonia can produce this picture. However, the signs of the loss of volume in the left lung along with the necrotizing airspace disease or pneumatoceles suggest that this is more likely staphylococcal pneumonia. Associated conditions include septic arthritis, endocarditis, and brain abscess. Reye syndrome is unlikely in an adult and is not an applicable choice here.

Unilateral Complete Opacification

146 Chest Radiology

DIRECTIONS: For each item below, match the scenario with the appropriate x-ray.

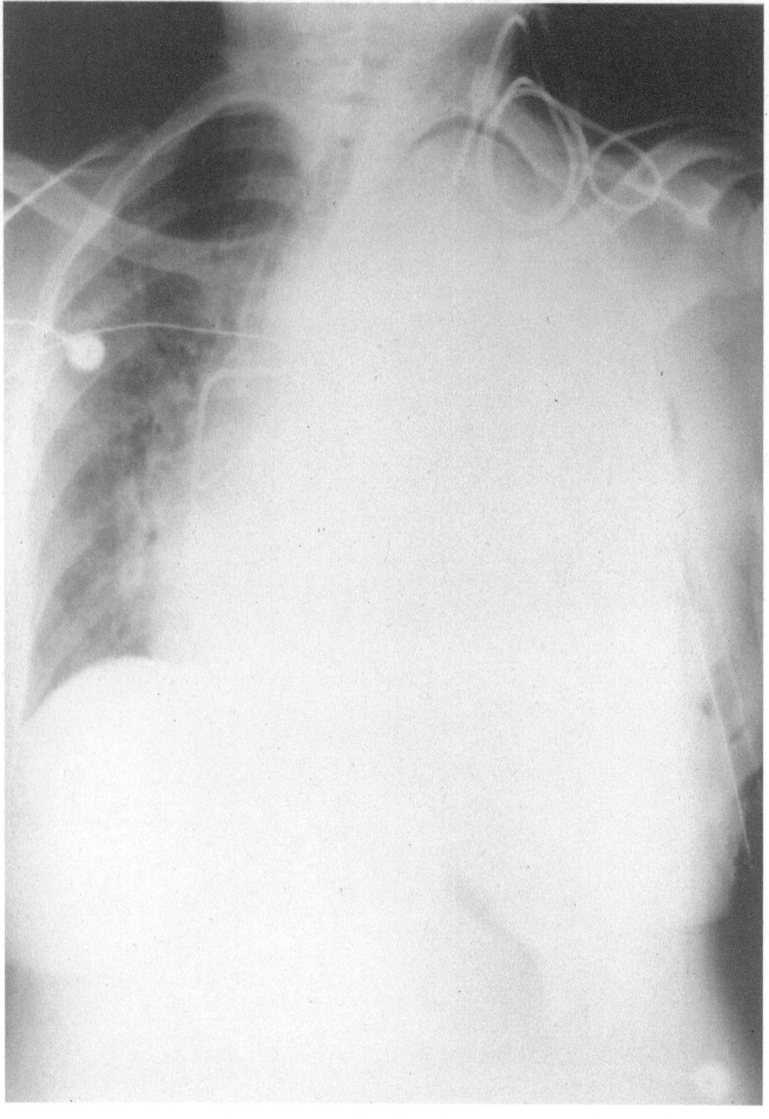

Fig. 43

Unilateral Complete Opacification 147

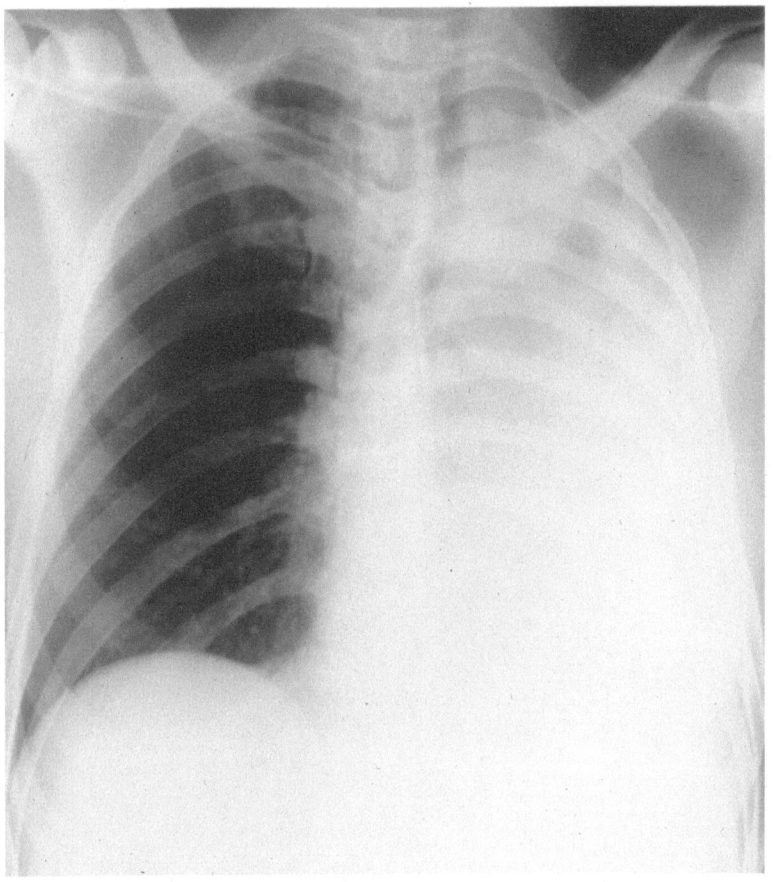

Fig. 44

148 Chest Radiology

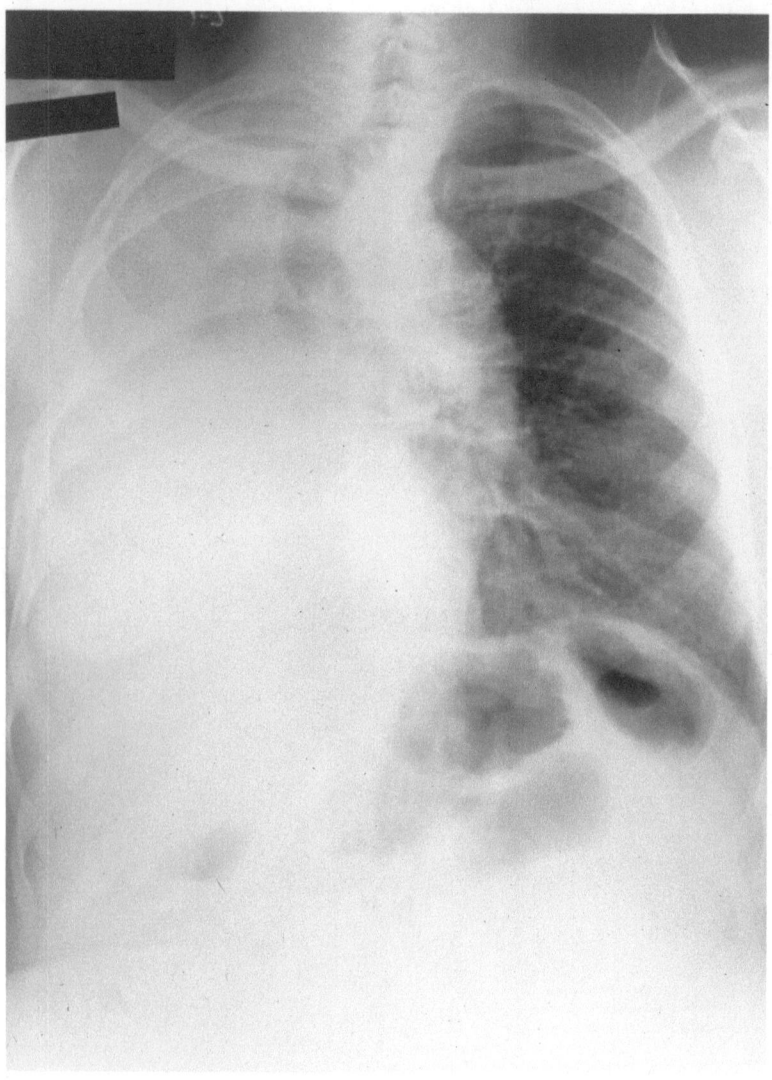

Fig. 45

Unilateral Complete Opacification   Answers   149

78. A 45-year-old man is admitted with progressive shortness of breath. On exam he has stony dullness to percussion. Breath sounds are absent in the left lung field. Which of the above chest x-rays is most likely to belong to this patient?
 a. Fig. 43
 b. Fig. 44
 c. Fig. 45

79. A 78-year-old man is admitted from a nursing home with a history of progressive dyspnea. On exam he is in moderate distress; lung exam reveals decreased breath sounds in the left lung field with dullness to percussion in the left hemithorax. Which of the above chest x-rays is most likely to belong to this patient?
 a. Fig. 43
 b. Fig. 44
 c. Fig. 45

80. A 70-year-old male smoker with a history of COPD is evaluated for hemotypsis. He has a history of asbestos exposure. On examination he has a scar on the right side of the thorax posterolaterally; bronchial breath sounds are heard in the right upper lung zone anteriorly with absent breath sounds in the right base. Diffuse rhonchi/wheezes are heard on the left side. Which of the above chest x-rays is most likely to belong to this patient?
 a. Fig. 43
 b. Fig. 44
 c. Fig. 45

UNILATERAL COMPLETE OPACIFICATION

Answers

Description of X-rays in This Chapter

Figure 43. This is an anterior-posterior film with reasonable inflation of the right lung. The patient is not intubated, but the monitoring wires, right heart catheter, and chest tube suggest an intensive care setting. The heart with appropriately placed RHC is shifted to the right hemithorax. There is subcutaneous air surrounding the exit of the chest tubes with air at the apex of the left chest without an air-fluid level. The stomach shadow, which appears to contain air, is displaced downward and to the right. Pleural fluid is most likely to show complete opacification and a contralateral shift of the mediastinum. The apical air and the presence of a chest tube suggest the fluid is loculated and not being adequately drained.

Figure 44. A central line is present emphasizing the marked cardiac displacement into the left chest. The trachea is also markedly displaced leftward with only minimal right anterior oblique patient positioning. A homogeneous density occupies the entire left hemithorax, silhouetting the left cardiac border and the left diaphragm. The more radiographically opaque left lower thorax opacity is owing to the superimposed heart density, while the left upper thorax likely contains some anteriorly herniated right lung. The left main bronchus appears narrow.

Figure 45. The 4th posterior rib is absent. The trachea is displaced to the right and foreshortened consistent with a reduced right-sided thoracic space. The heart and left hilum are markedly shifted to the right, with the cardiac apex barely visible in the left chest. The right hemithorax consists of a homogeneous opacity greater at the base due to the displaced cardiac density. There is a relative radiolucency lining the right paraspinal region and hilum due to anterior herniation of the left lung past the midline.

General Discussion

A pneumonectomy is typically performed through the posterior lateral thoracotomy for resection of bronchogenic carcinoma. The postpneumonectomy pleural space slowly accumulates serosangineous fluid, and an air-fluid level may persist for months. Increased air in the hemithorax signals the development of a bronchopleural fistula. Eventually the space completely fills with fluid, and the hemithorax decreases in size as the fluid is absorbed and organization progresses. The thorax decreases in size with primarily inward displacement of the chest wall. However, the remaining space is filled by a shift in the surrounding mediastinum and diaphragm. Hyperinflated contralateral lung compensates for the shift. Following left pneumonectomy, the mediastinum shifts so that the usual anterior and posterior orientation of the aortic arch is maintained. The right lung may herniate posteriorly or anteriorly. Following right pneumonectomy, the mediastinum rotates and the left lung herniates anteriorly. In general, the smaller the pneumonectomy space, the greater the herniation. Opacification of the hemothorax makes radiographic evaluation of new recurring cancer difficult.

Pulmonary atelectasis or collapse on chest radiograph is discussed in Chap. 9.

X-ray features of pleural effusion include opacity without air bronchograms, blunted costophrenic angles, a "meniscus" sign (further discussed in Chap. 12), or a complete opacification of the hemithorax. In the supine position, pleural fluid collects in the posterior medial hemithorax and the dependent portion, and presents as a diffuse opacity on the affected side. Such opacity without air bronchograms is diagnostic. Pleural effusions can also cause atelectasis of the underlying lung with displaced lower lobe collapse. A large pleural effusion may opacify the entire hemithorax, creating a mass effect and collapsing the lung with contralateral shift of the mediastinum. Air in the stomach may make the presence of effusion obvious because of diaphragmatic displacement on the left. The peak of the diaphragm is more laterally placed with a small subpulmonic effusion. Decubitus positioning confirms the effusion if it is mobile. Thoracostomy tubes are used to drain pleural collections of fluid if the effusion is symptomatic.

Specific Discussion

78. The answer is c. In this patient with a thoracotomy scar secondary to a right-sided pneumonectomy, the radiographic signs reveal ipsilateral shift of the mediastinum. The history and symptoms of COPD account for the physical signs noted in the left lung. The bronchial breath sounds heard on the right side anteriorly are due to transmitted sounds from the trachea.

79. The answer is b. This patient has signs of left-sided atelectasis probably due to an endobronchial obstruction or a mucus plug. Atelectasis is confirmed by the ipsilateral mediastinal shift on the CXR with a homogeneous opacity on the same side. The rib spaces are narrower than on the right and there are no rib changes suggesting a pneumonectomy or any surgery.

80. The answer is a. The physical signs and the chest radiograph are consistent with a massive left-sided pleural effusion. The contralateral mediastinal shift can also be seen secondary to a pleural or lung mass on the left side. However, masses of that degree are rare.

PLEURAL DISEASE

Pleural Disease

DIRECTIONS: Each item below contains a question or incomplete statement followed by suggested responses. Select the **one best** response to each question.

Items 81–82

A 60-year-old man, a lifetime resident of northern Louisiana, is referred with increasing cough, shortness of breath, and an abnormal chest radiograph. This patient has a past history of hypertension. On physical examination, he is afebrile with pulse 110 bpm; respirations 21/min; blood pressure 160/100 mm Hg. Other pertinent findings include S_3 and S_4 gallop, decreased breath sounds bilaterally, mild cardiomegaly, and pedal edema. Laboratory data: Hb 13 g/dL; Hct 39%; WBCs 10.0/µL; BUN 34 mg/dL; creatinine 1.2 mg/dL; sodium 121 mEq/L; potassium 4.0 mEq/L.

Chest x-rays are shown in Fig. 46.

81. What is the most likely diagnosis?

a. Bronchogenic CA
b. Round pneumonia
c. Neurofibroma
d. Interlobar effusion

82. What is the next management option?

a. Perform computed tomography of the chest
b. Start antibiotics
c. Begin vasodilator and diuretic therapy
d. Perform a bronchoscopy

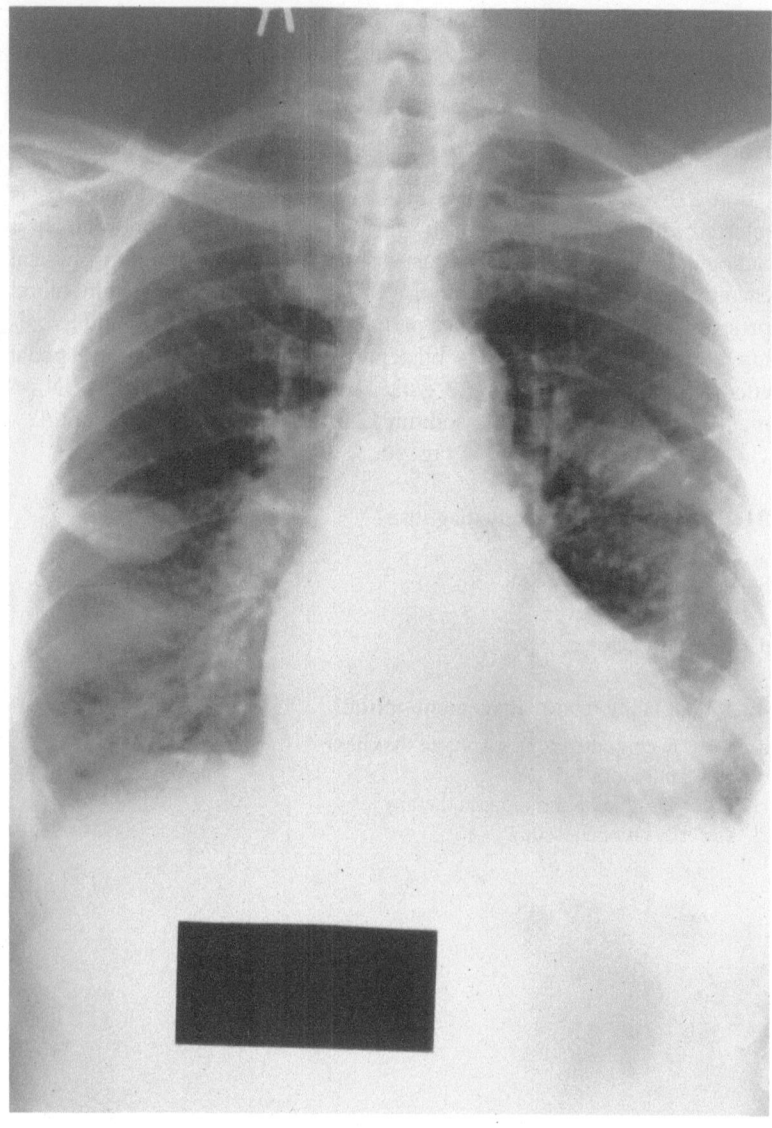

Fig. 46a

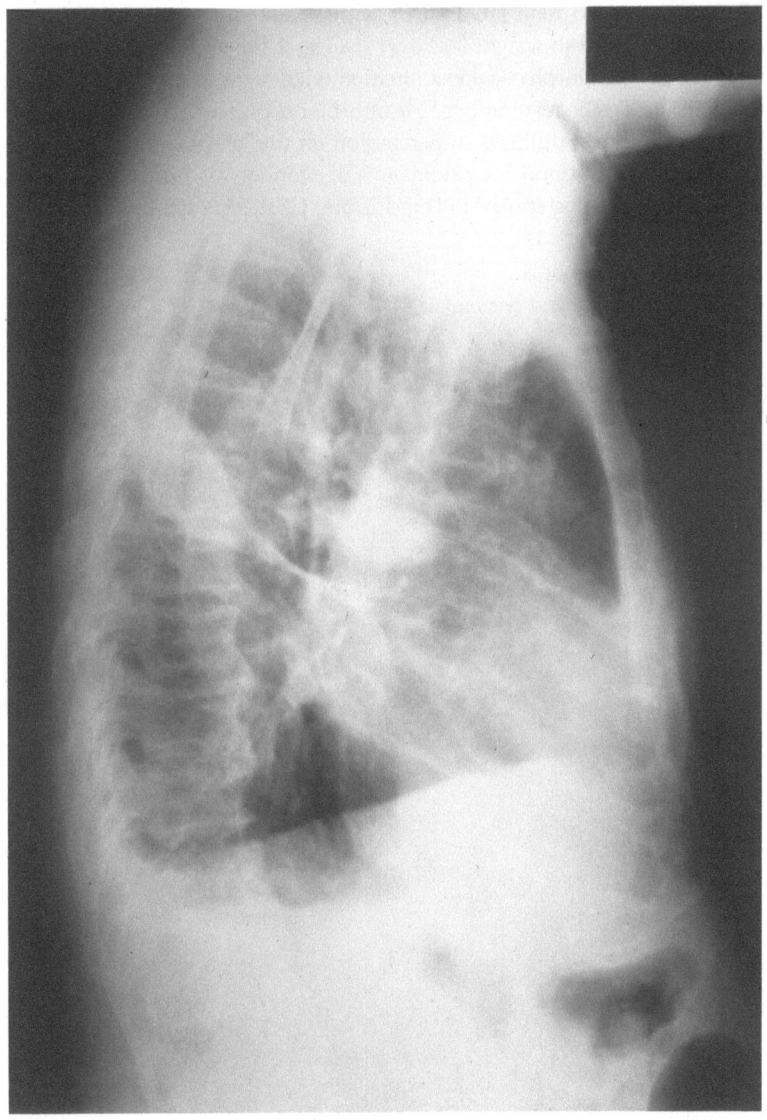

Fig. 46b

83. A 41-year-old man is admitted with severe shortness of breath. He complains of a 25-lb weight loss over the last 2 mo and occasional vomiting after meals. On physical examination, vital signs are: pulse 110 bpm; temperature 98°F; respirations 24/min; blood pressure 110/70 mm Hg. Pertinent findings: dullness to percussion on the left posterior chest with decreased breath sounds. A patchy area of egophony is heard over the left upper lung field posteriorly. PPD is 15 mm. CXR is shown in Fig. 47. The most likely diagnosis is

a. Aspiration pneumonia
b. Community-acquired pneumonia
c. Pleural effusion
d. Left lung atelectasis

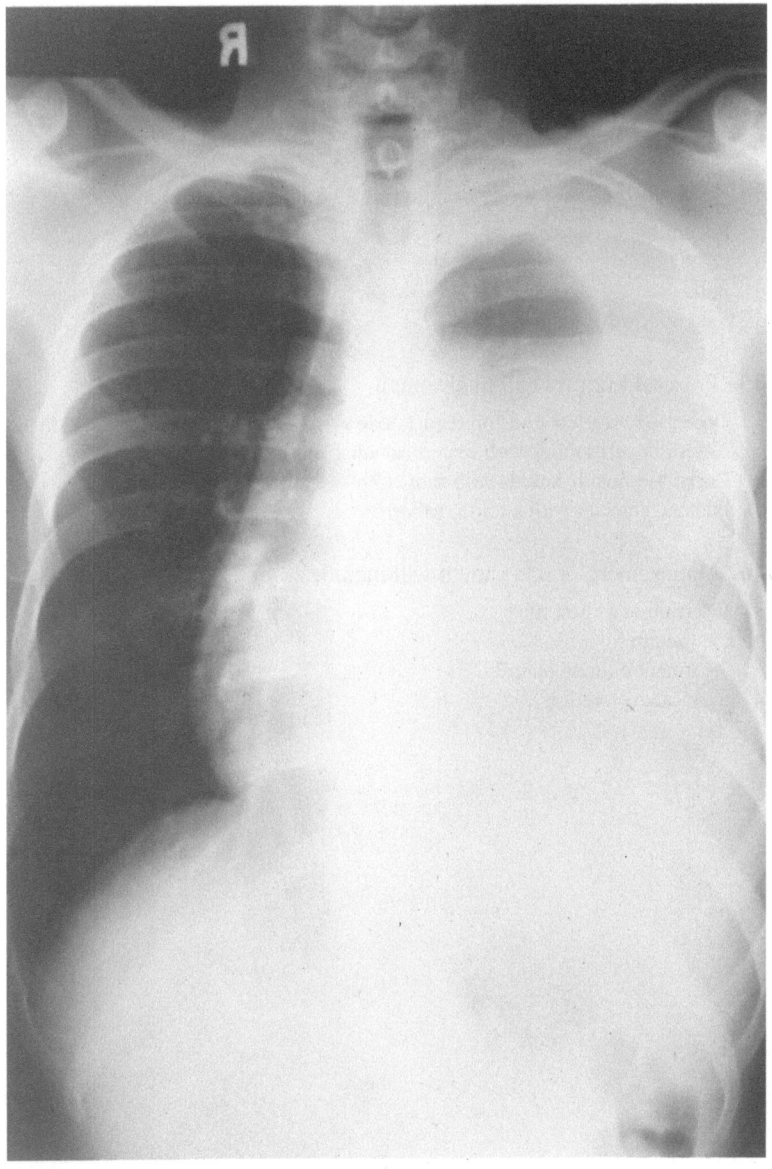

Fig. 47

Items 84–86

A 44-year-old man with a history of chronic bronchitis is admitted with severe shortness of breath and left-sided chest pain. CXR is shown in Fig. 48. EKG shows left ventricular strain.

84. What is the most likely diagnosis to explain the symptoms?
a. Pneumothorax
b. COPD
c. Bulla
d. Subendocardial infarct

85. Physical findings will likely entail
a. Decreased breath sounds on the left side with stony dullness on percussion
b. Absent breath sounds with hyperresonance on the left side
c. Decreased breath sounds with rhonchi bilaterally
d. Bilateral crackles with an S_3-S_4 gallop

86. Management of this patient will include
a. Insertion of a chest tube
b. Pleural tap
c. Treatment of heart failure
d. Surgical exploration

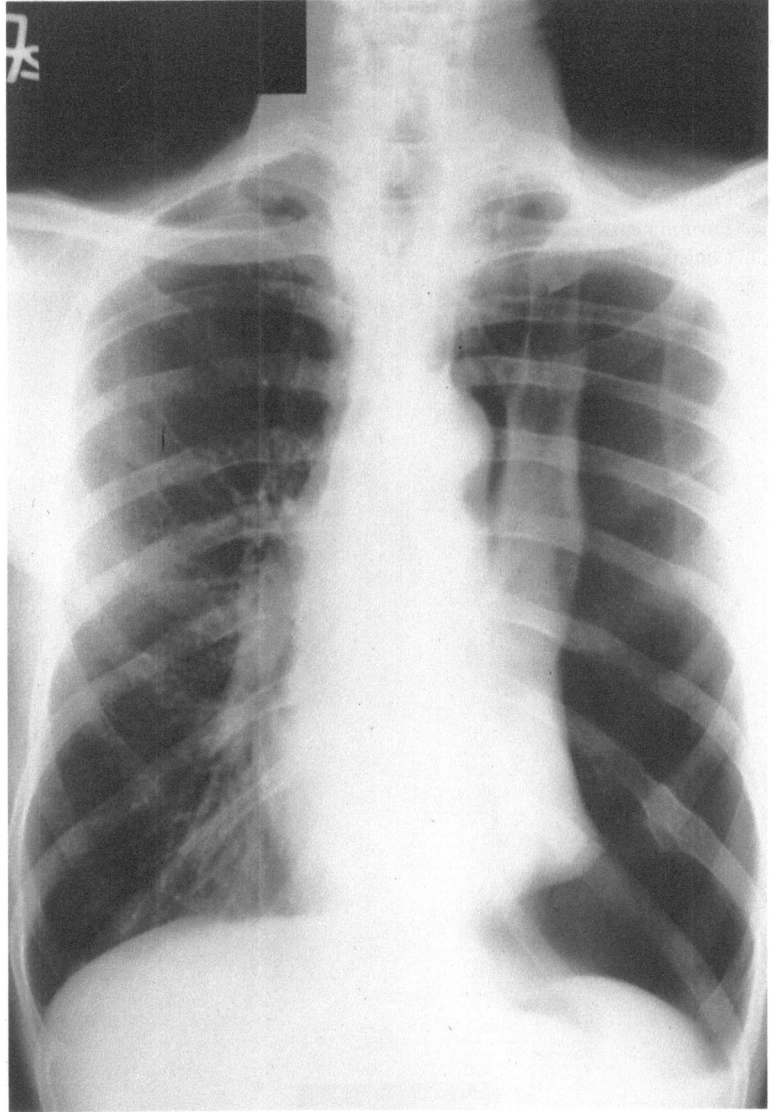

Fig. 48

87. A 60-year-old man is admitted for elective hernia repair. He has a 40-pack-per-year smoking history and worked as a construction worker for 20 years. He complains of shortness of breath and occasional blood-streaked sputum. His ECG shows lateral wall ischemia. The findings on his chest x-rays (Fig. 49) are due to

a. Chronic bronchitis
b. Empyema
c. Environmental occupational exposure
d. Congestive heart failure

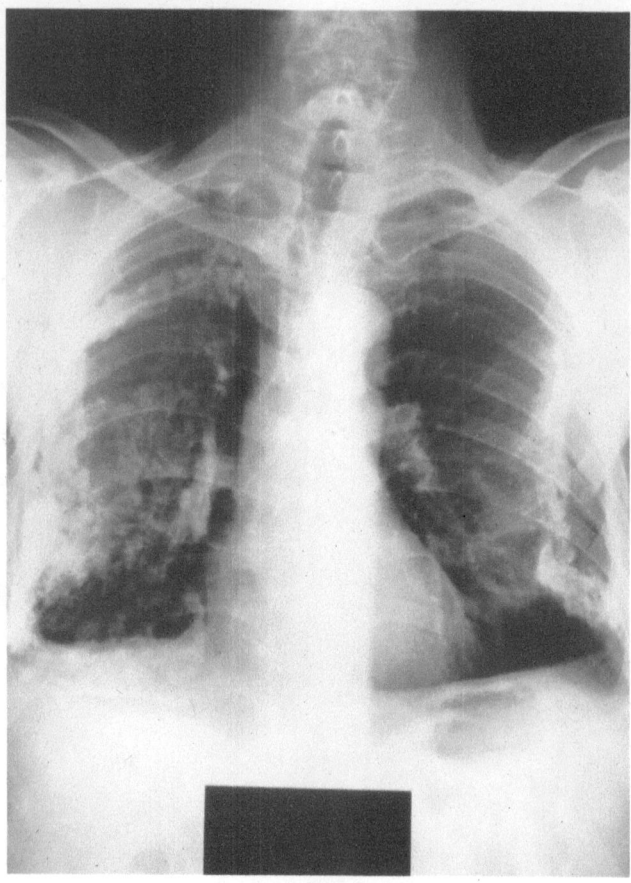

Fig. 49a

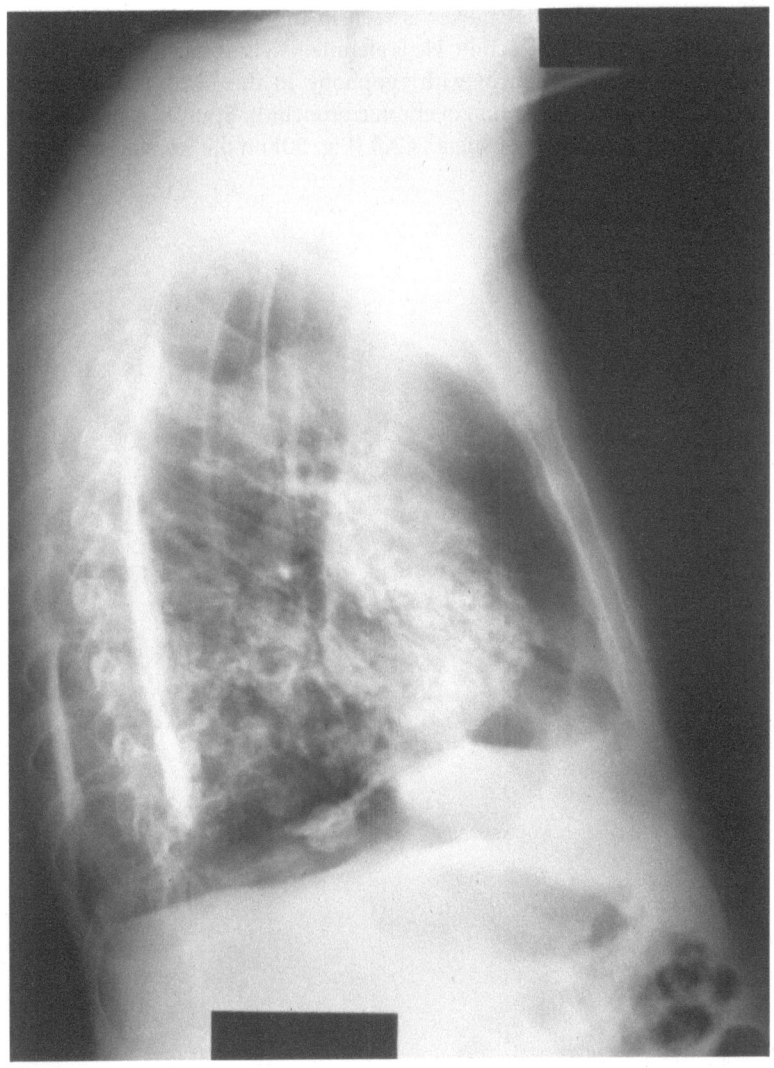

Fig. 49b

88. A 70-year-old male smoker is seen in the clinic with symptoms of cough and sputum production. He is afebrile. On lung exam, there are left-sided crackles and rhonchi with egophony in the LUL. The patient is treated for acute exacerbation of chronic bronchitis. Sputum is negative for AFB. The changes on the patient's CXR (Fig. 50) on the left side are due to

a. Chronic bronchitis
b. LUL pneumonia
c. Old granulomatous disease
d. Asbestos exposure

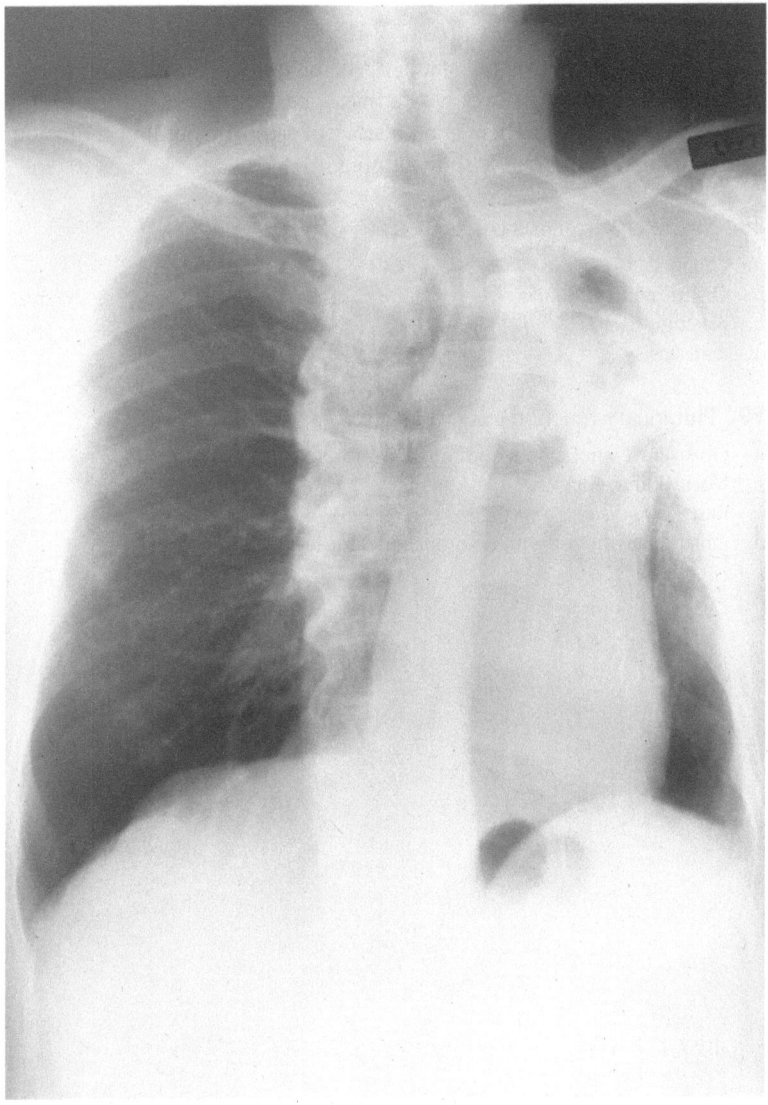

Fig. 50

Items 89–90

A 53-year-old female nonsmoker is being evaluated with symptoms of progressive shortness of breath. She has a past history of trauma to the right side of the chest. There is no history of asthma, sputum production, or recent chest pain. CXR is shown in Fig. 51.

89. The likely diagnosis is
 a. Calcified cyst
 b. Organized hemothorax
 c. Blastomycosis
 d. Asbestosis

90. Pulmonary function tests will show
 a. Obstructive limitation with bronchodilator response
 b. Normal lung volumes
 c. Restrictive disease
 d. Obstructive disease with no bronchodilator response

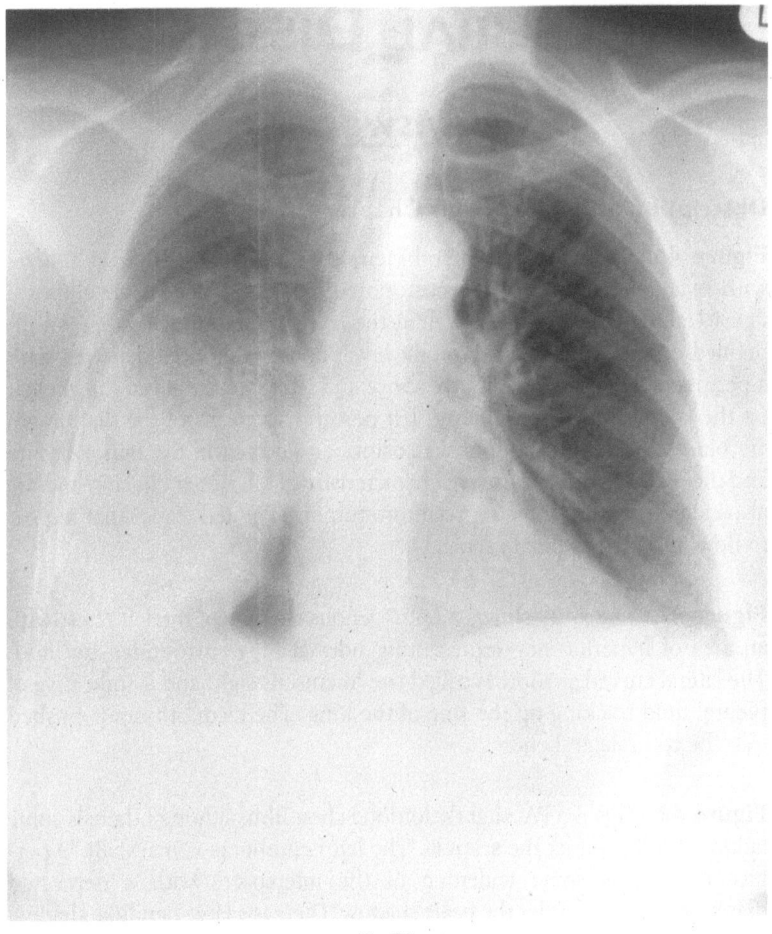

Fig. 51

PLEURAL DISEASE

Answers

Description of X-rays in This Chapter

Figure 46. These PA and lateral views reveal a large cardiac silhouette with bilateral blunting of the costophrenic angles. There is an elliptical density along the right chest wall at the level of the minor fissure. An ill-defined opacity appears in the right lower zone. Additional densities with a peripheral edge appear slightly above and lateral to the hilum on the left on the lateral film. The right and left posterior portions of the diaphragm are blunted. The three elliptical densities are located in the minor fissure and the major fissure. These are characteristic of interlobar effusion and are also called pseudotumors or phantom tumors. Pointed "tails" that appear to flow into the fissure are typical.

Figure 47. The x-ray shows a homogenous shadow of the left chest with an area of hyperlucency representing normal lung surrounded by fluid. The lateral curved shadow is called the "meniscus sign" and is indicative of pleural fluid tracking up the side of the lung. The mediastinum is pushed into the contralateral chest.

Figure 48. This is a PA, slightly lordotic chest film, although there is some failure to fully abduct the scapula. The left hemithorax is markedly hyperlucent; there is some widening of the interspaces with a depressed diaphragm and air under the heart shadow. There is a large bandlike shadow extending from the apex of the left lung down to the bottom of the heart with silhouetting of the left cardiac border. This represents a total lung collapse with atelectasis; however, some of the air totally surrounds the lung with hyperlucency around the aortic knob. Most pneumothoraces usually show a sharp edge differentiating the free air in the pleural space from the normal pulmonary parenchyma, with a line representing the pleural surfaces. In this particular case, because of marked collapse with circumferential air, one does not see the sharp line and observes bilateral edges, i.e., differences in contrast between a more radiodense and radiolucent background. The very sharp edge along the left heart border represents the contrast between the collapsed lung and the pleural space and is called the *visceral pleural line*. The chest wall appears irregular along the level of lateral 6th to 7th ribs, probably representing a rib fracture.

Figure 49. The PA roentgenogram shows a prominent trachea shadow minimally displaced to the right; there are very dense irregular shadows in both the left and right thorax, probably representing calcific pleural plaques. There are linear plaques of both parietal diaphragmatic surfaces as well. The lateral film of the same patient shows marked calcification in the right posterior sulcus from the top almost to the bottom of the lung; there is also heavy calcification along the lateral pleural surfaces and some calcification along the diaphragm, primarily on the right.

Figure 50. The PA view of the chest shows marked deviation of the trachea into the left hemithorax. The left main stem bronchus is pulled upward, and the left hilum is substantially elevated; the thin, radiodense lines coming from the hilum to the left lower chest are the pulled, stretched pulmonary arteries. There is substantial thickening of the lateral pleural wall, especially in the left upper lobe region. An inhomogeneous density in the left upper lobe region represents bronchiectasis and cystic changes of the destroyed left upper lobe.

Figure 51. There is a large, well-demarcated, calcified pleural-based opacity abutting the lateral chest occupying two-thirds of the left hemithorax. It has a rounded, intensely calcified inferior and medial border and thus suggests a pleural origin. The shadow is most consistent with a large, old organized hemothorax.

General Discussion

The chest x-ray features of pleural effusion include a homogeneous opacity without air bronchograms, blunted costophrenic angle, the "meniscus" sign, and complete or near-complete opacification of the hemithorax with contralateral mediastinal shift. Radiographically, blunting of the lateral costophrenic angle and preservation of the posterior angle almost always indicate scarring rather than effusion. The interface between the lung and the effusion is usually concave medially and is termed a *meniscus*. The meniscus sign is seen usually on upright PA and lateral films. A large pleural effusion may opacify the entire hemithorax, creating a mass effect and collapsing the lung with contralateral shifting of the mediastinum. Pleural fluid may collect in the subpleural location and a subpulmonic effusion may be overlooked because it mimics elevation of the hemidiaphragm. Air in the stomach may make the presence of effusion apparent on the left. A lateral peak of the diaphragm often indicates the presence of subpulmonic effusion. Decubitus positioning confirms the effusion if it is mobile. Fluid located within the fissure may produce a pseudotumor, which can simulate an intrapulmonary mass in one or more projections. However, the characteristic elliptical shadow indicates the true nature of the density. A sharp horizontal interface indicates a fluid level and is diagnostic for a hydropneumothorax. Lateral decubitus examination is the more sensitive test to detect fluid and can detect as much as 10 cc of fluid. Small effusions can also be seen on CT scan. In a supine position, pleural fluid collects in the posterior medial hemothorax and the dependent portion of the chest, and may present as a diffuse opacity on the affected side in the anteroposterior projection. Such opacity without air bronchograms is diagnostic. Pleural effusions can also cause atelectasis of the underlying lung with collapse of the displaced lower lobe. About 25 cc of fluid can cause progressive flattening of the diaphragm and inversion; yet it does not produce blunting of the left costophrenic angle on the PA view. Blunting of the costophrenic angle on the PA view is seen when about 200 cc of fluid has collected. Blunting of the posterior costophrenic angle on the lateral view can be seen with as little as 50 cc of fluid collection.

Pleural effusions are the most common pleural pathology. Fluid accumulates when lymphatic absorption is impaired. The most common causes of pleural effusion include congestive heart failure, pneumonia, pulmonary embolism, and tumor. Clinically, patients may have dyspnea or chest pain. Effusions can easily obscure a significant underlying pathology. Effusions are classified as transudates or exudates according to their biochemical composition. Transudates are the results of increased hydrostatic pressure or decreased colloidal osmotic pressure and usually result from systemic causes such as congestive heart failure or hyperketonemic states such as cirrhosis. Transudates are usually homogeneous with near-water attenuation on CT and are often bilateral. Particularly, they have a low protein count, low LDH, low protein fluid–to–serum protein ratio, and low fluid–to–serum LDH ratio. Exudates are usually a result of a local inflammatory process involving the pleura due to the infection or tumor. The incidence of parapneumonic pleural effusion is dependent upon the organism; 10% of pneumonias caused by pneumococci can cause parapneumonic effusion. Fifty percent of pneumonias caused by staphylococci can cause effusion. Exudates have increased protein, increased LDH, and increased ratios. Bilateral effusions are usually transudates. Unilateral effusions are most often exudates; left-sided effusions occur due to rupture of the esophagus, dissecting aneurysm, or traumatic injury to the aorta. Pancreatitis also typically leads to left-sided effusion. Pleural thickening and enhancement on CT usually indicates an exudate. Pleural fluid with an inhomogeneous appearance suggests a hemothorax; its causes include trauma, malignancy, embolism, and, rarely, pleural endometriosis. Imaging is helpful, but thoracentesis is the mainstay in the diagnosis because the composition of the fluid suggests its etiology. *Chylothorax* refers to effusion containing lymphatic fluid, which has high triglyceride content. Fifty percent of chylothoraces are related to tumors such as lymphoma. Resection and transection of the lower thoracic duct occur during surgery or after trauma. An empyema is most likely a result of infected parapneumonic effusion. It can occur as a complication of trauma, septic infarction, and other infectious process. An empyema generally has a smooth wall and conforms to the pleural space. Thoracostomy tubes or thoracotomy are used to drain pleural collections of fluid.

Specific Discussion

81–82. The answers are 81-d, 82-c. This patient presented with symptoms and signs of congestive heart failure. The presence of cardiomegaly, hilar congestion, and interlobar pleural effusion, as noted in the description of the x-rays, is essentially diagnostic of heart failure. Fluid resolves with appropriate therapy but may recur in the same area with subsequent bouts of CHF. There is no posterior mediastinal mass or other skin manifestations that could accompany a neurofibroma. The clinical picture is inconsistent with pneumonia, and the multiple opacities in the location of the fissures make bronchogenic carcinoma unlikely.

83. The answer is c. This patient complained of shortness of breath with physical signs of a left-sided pleural effusion. This is confirmed by the chest x-ray. The clinical presentation in this afebrile patient without any airspace disease makes community-acquired pneumonia unlikely. Atelectasis of the left lung due to mucus plugging or aspiration would produce a homogenous opacity with ipsilateral shift of the mediastinum. In this case the meniscus sign and the contralateral mediastinal shift make the diagnosis of pleural effusion very likely.

84–86. The answers are 84-a, 85-b, 86-a. The acute onset of severe shortness of breath and left-sided chest pain suggests concurrent pleural disease as part of the differential diagnosis. This is confirmed by the chest x-ray showing a left-sided pneumothorax. Patients with COPD and/or bullous disease have chronic symptoms. With an acute exacerbation of COPD, the chest x-ray is helpful in distinguishing a pneumothorax vs. pneumonia. On physical exam, patients with pneumothorax present with absent breath sounds and hyperresonance on the side of the pneumothorax. The other physical findings mentioned are not characteristic of pneumothorax. Management of a symptomatic patient with a large pneumothorax is by insertion of a chest tube.

87. The answer is c. The chest x-ray shows dense bilateral pleural plaques and diaphragmatic calcification characteristic of asbestos-related disease. Pleural plaques, malignant mesothelioma, asbestosis, and lung cancer occur after a long latency period. Asbestos-related pleural effusions are often bloody, exudative, and difficult to differentiate from those caused by trauma, neoplasm, or thromboembolic disease. Diagnosis is based on history of occupational exposure and exclusion of other causes. Chronic bronchitis is a clinical diagnosis, and the chest radiograph and clinical picture are not suggestive of CHF. Empyema presents as a pleural effusion or a loculated pleural-based opacity and not with diffuse bilateral calcification.

88. The answer is c. Although the clinical symptoms are suggestive of chronic bronchitis, the chest radiograph suggests old, inactive granulomatous disease like TB, with pleural-based opacity and loss of volume. Left upper lobe pneumonia does not cause loss of volume unless it is secondary to a necrotizing process.

89–90. The answers are 89-b, 90-c. The calcified and organized pleural-based opacity is consistent with an old hemothorax secondary to previous trauma. The pulmonary functions in this case would show restrictive limitation due to fibrosis of the pleural space and decreased lung compliance.

Pulmonary Vascular Disease

DIRECTIONS: Each item below contains a question or incomplete statement followed by suggested responses. Select the **one best** response to each question.

Items 91–92

A 29-year-old man is seen in the chest clinic. A week ago he was seen in the ER with symptoms of headache, fever, and metallic taste in his mouth. He denied any specific respiratory symptoms. It was noted in the ER record that he had a history of substance abuse. His physical exam was normal except for needle tracks in his right arm. At that time, before a complete evaluation was done, he left the ER against medical advice. A CXR done in the ER is retrieved (Fig. 52). The patient is currently asymptomatic and came to the clinic because he wanted a general checkup.

91. The feature that was positive in this patient's review of systems and history that is most helpful in reaching the diagnosis is
a. Recent contact with active TB
b. Occupational exposure to chicken farming
c. Seizure disorder
d. History of intravenous substance abuse

92. Based on the chest x-ray, the most likely diagnosis is
a. Primary TB
b. Silicosis
c. Pulmonary embolization of metallic particles
d. Sarcoidosis

Pulmonary Vascular Disease 175

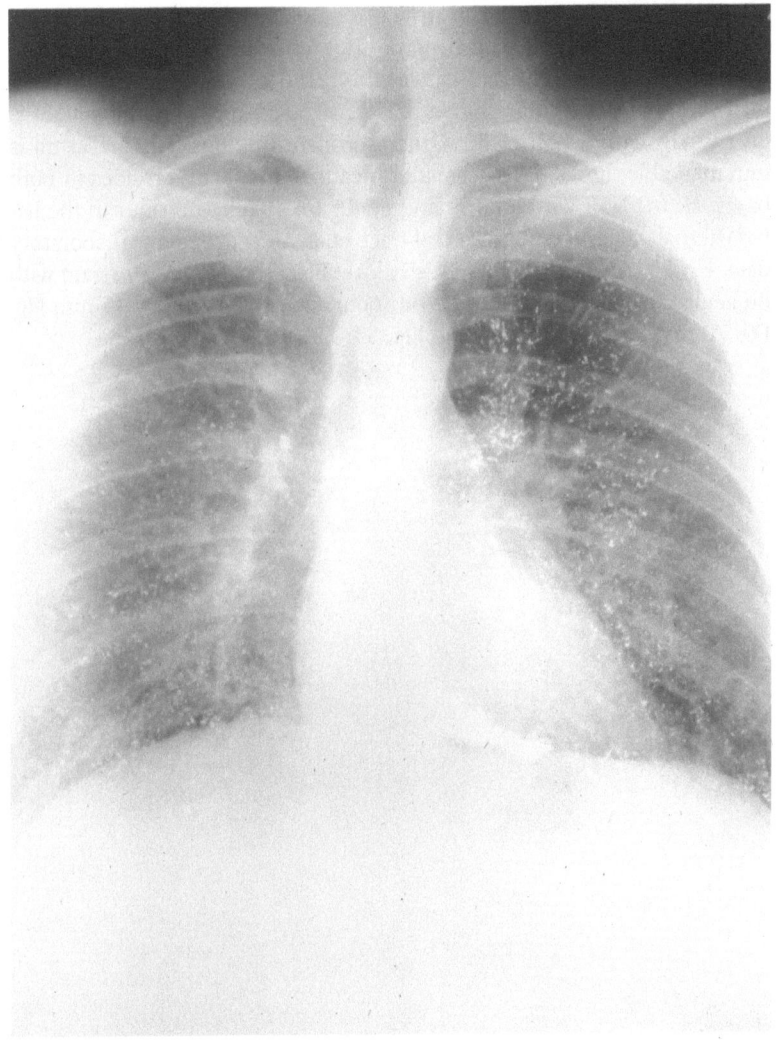

Fig. 52

93. A 34-year-old female cab driver, a smoker, is admitted with acute shortness of breath and mild hemoptysis. Her review of systems is otherwise unremarkable. Physical examination: pulse 100 bpm; temperature 99°F; respirations 21/min; blood pressure 160/84 mm Hg. The patient is overweight with a BMI of 30. Other pertinent findings: HEENT exam is unremarkable; lungs have decreased breath sounds with crackles in both bases. Heart: NSR with loud P_2 and grade 2/6 systolic murmur in the left parasternal area. Extremities reveal trace bilateral pedal edema. Laboratory data: Hb 15 g/dL; Hct 45%; WBCs 7.0/µL. EKG shows mild LV strain with no acute current of injury. ABGs on room air: pH 7.38; P_{CO_2} 45 mm Hg; P_{O_2} 70 mm Hg. CXR is shown in Fig. 53. The likely diagnosis is

a. Mycoplasma/atypical pneumonia
b. Obstructive sleep apnea
c. Chronic bronchitis
d. Pulmonary embolism

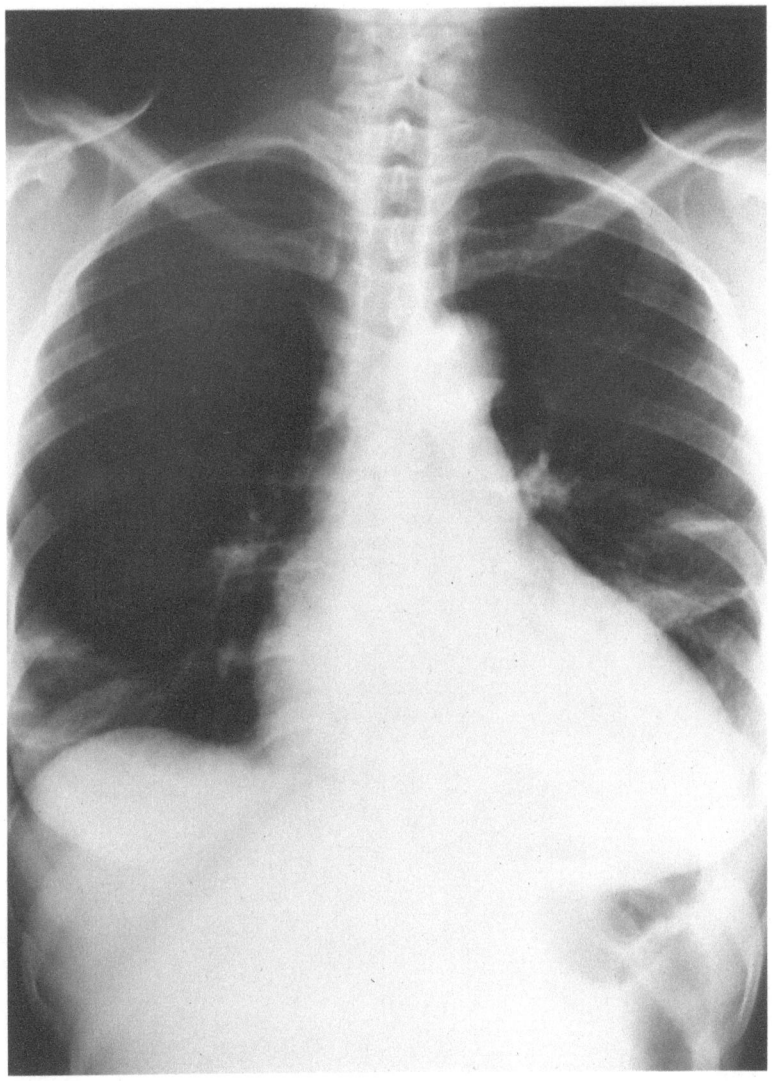

Fig. 53

Notes

Items 94–95

A 28-year-old G1, P0 26-wk pregnant woman is seen in the OB clinic. She has a past history of bronchial asthma that has been well controlled for the last year by inhaled steroids. She states that she has noted increasing shortness of breath for the last 3 days. On examination, she appears tachypneic and moderately uncomfortable. On physical examination, she has a pulse of 110 bpm; normal temperature; respirations 32/min; blood pressure 160/90 mm Hg. Heart exam: NSR without any gallop. A grade 2/6 systolic murmur in the pulmonic area is heard. Lung exam is clear to auscultation; abdomen exam confirms a 26-wk gravid uterus. Laboratory data: Hb 12 g/dL; Hct 36%; WBCs 7.0/µL with normal differential; BUN 23 mg/dL; creatinine 0.9 mg/dL; sodium 136 mEq/L; potassium 4.2 mEq/l. ABGs on room air: pH 7.34; P_{CO_2} 34 mm Hg; P_{O_2} 68 mm Hg. PEFR 450 L/min. Chest x-rays are shown in Fig. 54.

94. The most likely diagnosis is
a. Acute anxiety
b. Pulmonary embolism
c. Acute exacerbation of bronchial asthma
d. High-output heart failure

95. A further test that would be helpful to reach a diagnosis is
a. Pulmonary function test
b. Methacholine bronchoprovocation challenge test
c. Ventilation-perfusion (V/Q) scan
d. Six-minute exercise walk test

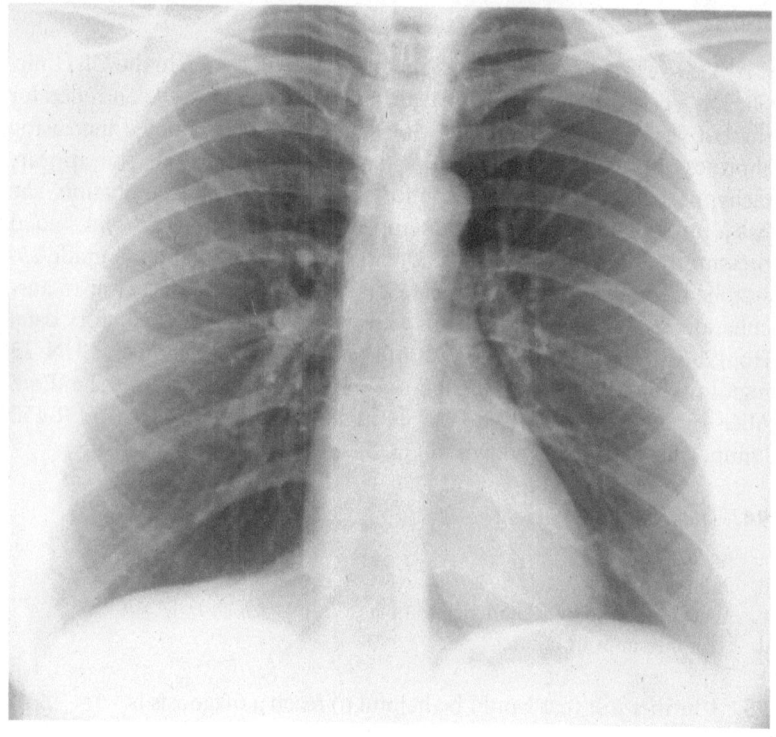

Fig. 54a

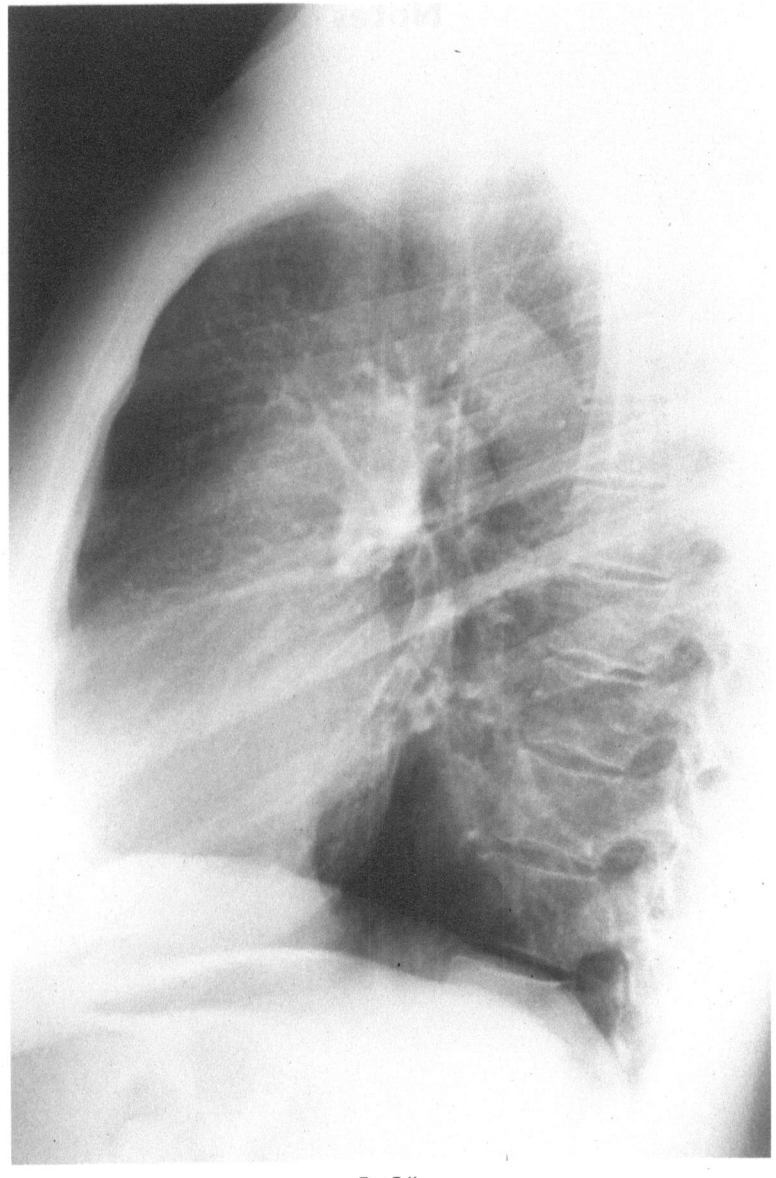

Fig. 54b

Notes

Items 96–97

A 24-year-old female graduate student reports increasing shortness of breath with exercise and has recently noticed dyspnea on mild activity. One day before presenting at the office, she experienced sudden loss of consciousness while shopping at a grocery store. On physical examination, vital signs are: pulse 88 bpm; temperature 97.8°F; respirations 18/min; blood pressure 100/70 mm Hg. BMI is 34. ABGs on RA: pH 7.43; P_{CO_2} 36 mm Hg; P_{O_2} 87 mm Hg. Chest x-rays are shown in Fig. 55.

96. The clinical and chest radiographic diagnosis may be commonly associated with

a. A loud A_2 on cardiac auscultation
b. Right arm swelling
c. Rib notching
d. A loud P_2 on cardiac auscultation

97. A further diagnostic test that will be specifically helpful to confirm the diagnosis is

a. Right heart catheterization
b. Bronchoscopy
c. Mediastinoscopy
d. V/Q scan

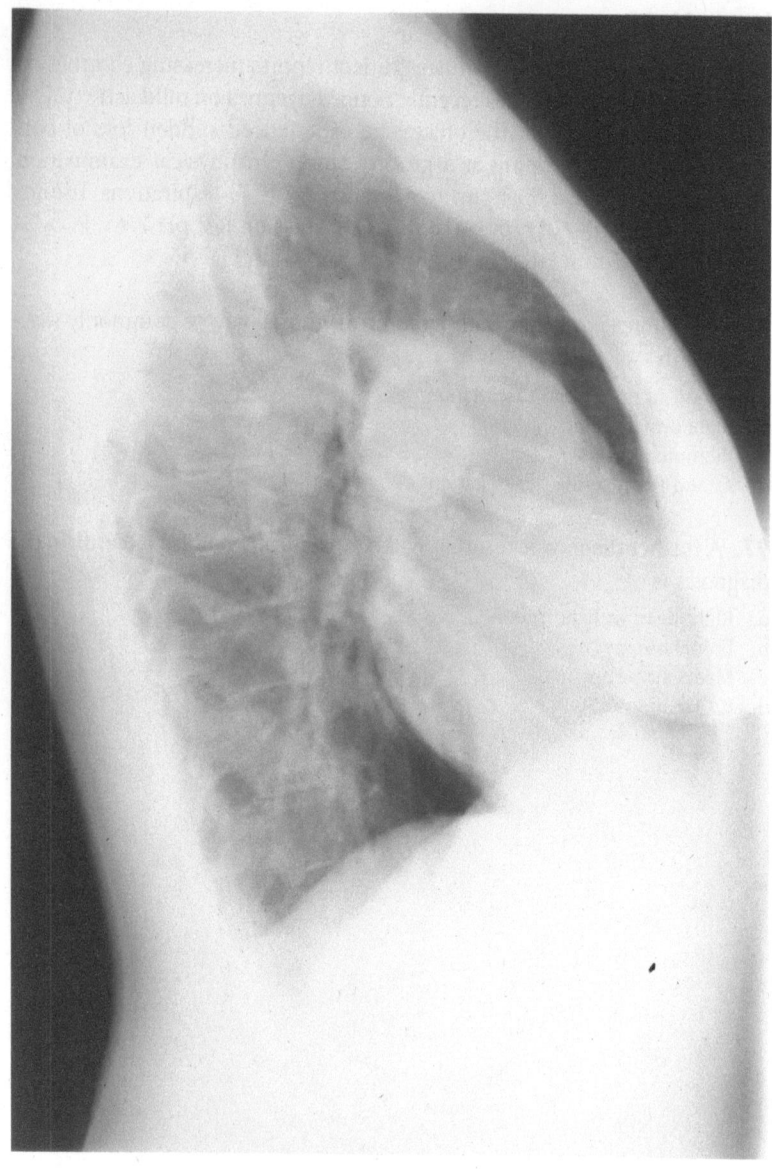

Fig. 55a

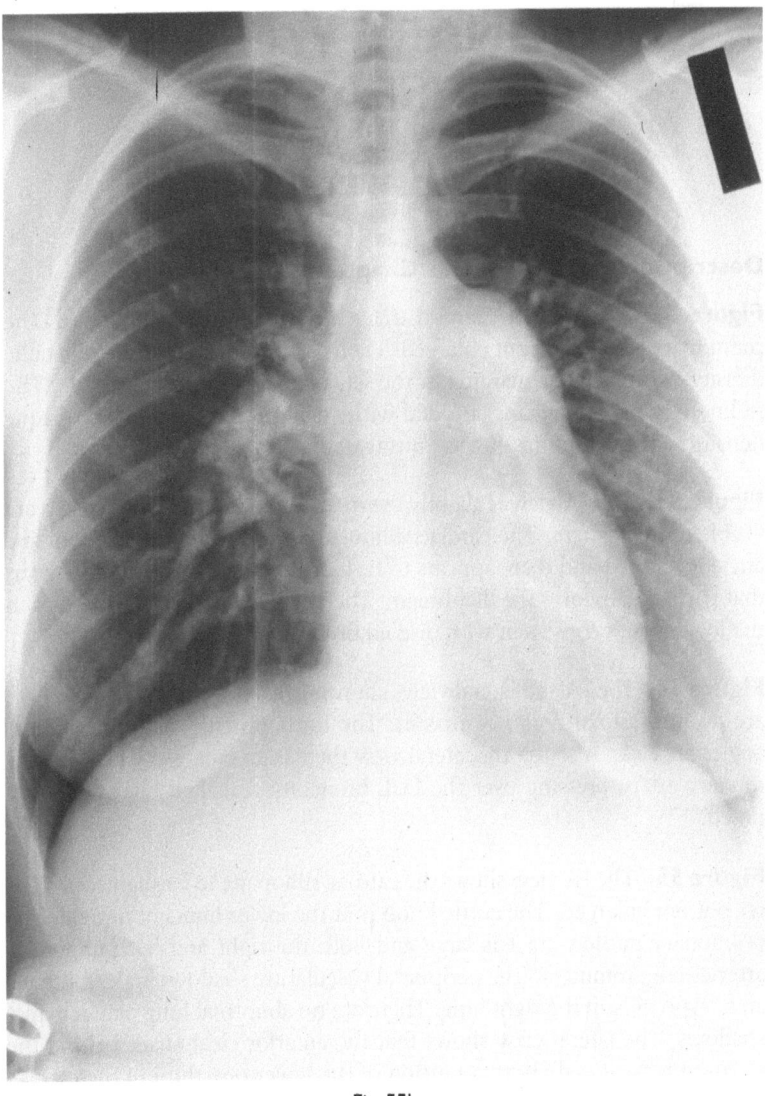

Fig. 55b

PULMONARY VASCULAR DISEASE

Answers

Description of X-rays in This Chapter

Figure 52. The PA view demonstrates a normal cardiac silhouette. The pulmonary arteries are not enlarged. There is an elongated opaque metallic density with irregular margins in the left medial costophrenic angle. The pulmonary parenchyma is studded with small nodular and linear opaque densities. These findings suggest intravascular embolization.

Figure 53. The PA view is slightly overpenetrated. Lumbar interspaces are visible in this patient. The cardiac silhouette is large. The left costophrenic angle is blunted and there appears to be increased density behind the heart that partially obscures the diaphragm. There are bilateral linear opacities in the lower zones consistent with discoid or linear atelectasis.

Figure 54. The PA and lateral views show normal lung parenchyma. There are no mediastinal nodes or masses. The cardiophrenic and costophrenic angles are clear. Also, on the lateral view there is an enlarged left main pulmonary artery pressing over the LUL bronchus. Calcified hilar nodes are noted.

Figure 55. The PA view shows the cardiac silhouette to be slightly off center but not enlarged. The aortic knob is at the lower limits of normal. The pulmonary outflow tract is large and both the right and left pulmonary arteries are prominent. The peripheral vasculature shadows appear attenuated, especially in the right lung. There are no abnormal lung parenchymal shadows. The lateral view shows that the anterior clear space behind the sternum is occupied above a portion of the lower one-third of the cardiac shadow. The truncus of the right pulmonary artery seen in front of the trachea is very large and the left main pulmonary artery coursing over the left upper lobe bronchus is greater than 16 mm. These findings are consistent with pulmonary arterial hypertension.

General Discussion

An increase in pulmonary artery pressure is called *pulmonary hypertension*. The various mechanisms of this increase include: (1) increase in left atrial pressure, as seen in mitral stenosis and left ventricular failure. This is further discussed in Chap. 15. (2) Increase in pulmonary blood flow, as occurs in congenital heart disease and left-to-right septal defects. Initially this causes no structural distortion in the vascular bed, since capillary distensibility and recruitment compensates for this increased pressure. Later, however, sustained increased pressure causes changes in small vessels with development of right-to-left shunt. (3) Increased pulmonary vascular resistance—the most common cause of cor pulmonale. This may be due to alveolar hypoxia, as seen in COPD, and is called *secondary pulmonary hypertension*. It is related to release of mediators such as serotonin and catecholamines. In pulmonary thromboembolic disease, the vessels are obstructed by thrombi or circulating cells, as seen in fat or air embolism. Further, pulmonary hypertension can occur when the capillary bed is obliterated as in pulmonary fibrosis or veno-occlusive disease. In some cases, several pathogeneses contribute to the elevated pressure at the same time. Primary pulmonary hypertension is defined as a disorder of unknown or undetermined cause and results from smooth muscle hyperplasia of small pulmonary arteries. The chest radiograph presentations of the above histological and pathologic entities are variable and will be discussed in the section below.

Specific Discussion

91–92. The answers are 91-d, 92-c. The inhalation, ingestion, or injection of mercury can produce toxicity, and the clinical scenario described is of an individual who has a history of intravenous substance abuse. The symptoms of headache, fever, and metallic taste in the mouth may follow intravenous injection of mercury. In severe cases, dyspnea, chest pain, and respiratory failure may develop. Metallic mercury can be introduced through an IV site. Foreign body granulomas may form in the lung without any systemic toxicity or demonstrable damage of the pulmonary vascular bed. CXR changes with metallic densities and spherules may remain for many years. The spherical shape of the mercury droplets can be differentiated from shrapnel, which has angular margins, and lymphangiographic dye, which presents as a diffuse haze. Barium and bronchographic contrast material produce a more linear opacity. Other forms of granulomas or inhalation exposure do not produce these chest radiograph changes.

93. The answer is d. Mycoplasma or atypical pneumonia may present with a similar radiographic picture, but in the absence of an acute febrile illness, that diagnosis seems unlikely. Chronic bronchitis is a clinical diagnosis and is defined per ATS criteria as a history of chronic sputum production for most of the days in a 3-mo period for at least two successive years. The chest x-ray may show large pulmonary vessels if there is longstanding cor pulmonale and generally does not show any focal opacities. Although the patient is obese and 60% of patients with obstructive sleep apnea (OSA) are overweight, there is no history of hypersomnolence, sleep fragmentation, sleep disorder, or other clinical evidence of sleep apnea syndrome. The clinical scenario presented is suggestive of pulmonary embolism. The physical exam suggesting bilateral atelectasis and the chest radiograph depicting those changes and representing congestive atelectasis are consistent with that diagnosis.

94–95. The answers are 94-b, 95-c. This is a classic example of a clinical scenario with a high likelihood of pulmonary embolism in a high-risk patient. The chest radiograph is often unimpressive or normal, as in this case. However, congestive atelectasis, as mentioned in the previous question, moderate bloody pleural effusion, and nodular or patchy infiltrates can be seen. In some cases unilateral oligemia (Westermark sign) is recognized. *Hampton's hump* is a term used to define pulmonary lobules filled with blood. These are triangular pleural-based infiltrates with their apex toward the hilum. The increased alveolar arterial gradient seen on the arterial blood gas study suggests a ventilation-perfusion (V/Q) mismatch and rules out an acute anxiety state as the cause of the symptoms. Although the patient has a history of bronchial asthma, the lung exam reveals no wheezing or expiratory prolongation and symptoms have been well controlled. Peak flows are satisfactory and hence an acute asthmatic attack is unlikely. With a hemoglobin level of 12 g/dL and no clinical evidence of heart failure, a diagnosis of high-output heart failure is incorrect. The clinical diagnosis of pulmonary embolism warrants further diagnostic steps. A V/Q scan would be most helpful in reaching a diagnosis, especially in this case with a normal CXR. Other tests to assess respiratory function or exercise-induced hypoxemia would be inappropriate in this clinical setting.

96–97. The answers are 96-a, 97-a. The chest x-ray shows large pulmonary arteries, and this, coupled with the clinical scenario, is consistent with primary pulmonary hypertension (PPH). As mentioned in the general discussion, this entity is due to an unknown cause. The physical sign most likely to be present would be a loud P_2, and right heart catheterization would confirm the high pulmonary artery (PA) pressures. Patients with PPH may give a history of syncopal episodes. A loud A_2 is heard in systemic hypertension, and rib notching is classically seen on the x-ray in coarctation of the aorta. Right arm swelling is seen with either a localized vascular or lymphatic obstruction such as postradiation, malignancy, or superior vena cava syndrome. This patient does not exhibit any of these signs. Since the hilar shadows are of vascular nature, mediastinoscopy or bronchoscopy would not be indicated and in fact may be dangerous if PA pressures are very high.

MEDIASTINAL COMPARTMENTS

DIRECTIONS: Each item below contains a question or incomplete statement followed by suggested responses. Select the **one best** response to each question.

Items 98–100

A 70-year-old is admitted from a nursing home with fever and mental status changes. On physical examination, vital signs are: pulse 114 bpm; temperature 102°F; respirations 26/min; blood pressure 100/60 mm Hg. General exam: delirious and confused. Pertinent findings: HEENT—pupils equal and reactive; neck exam—right carotid bruit; soft tissue swelling; lungs—harsh bronchial breath sounds in the anterior chest upper zone bilaterally, no egophony or crackles; heart—tachycardia, NSR, no murmurs, no visible pulsation. Laboratory data: Hb 11 g/dL; Hct 33%; WBCs 19,000/µL; differential 90% PMNs with 5% bands; BUN 40 mg/dL; creatinine 1.3 mg/dL; sodium 129 mEq/L; potassium 3.1 mEq/L. Urinalysis: 3+ bacteria. Thyroid function tests are normal. ABGs on room air: pH 7.34; P_{CO_2} 30 mm Hg; P_{O_2} 65 mm Hg. Chest radiograph is shown below in Fig. 56.

98. What is the CXR abnormality most likely to be?
a. Substernal goiter
b. Superior vena cava syndrome
c. Non-Hodgkin's lymphoma
d. Carotid aneurysm

99. While treating for presumed urosepsis, what is the next management option in relation to the chest x-ray abnormality?
a. Aortogram
b. Radiation treatment
c. CT scan of neck
d. Needle biopsy of thyroid

100. The flow volume loop of this patient will show
a. Reversible obstructive ventilatory impairment
b. Restrictive pattern
c. Irreversible obstructive ventilatory impairment
d. Fixed obstruction

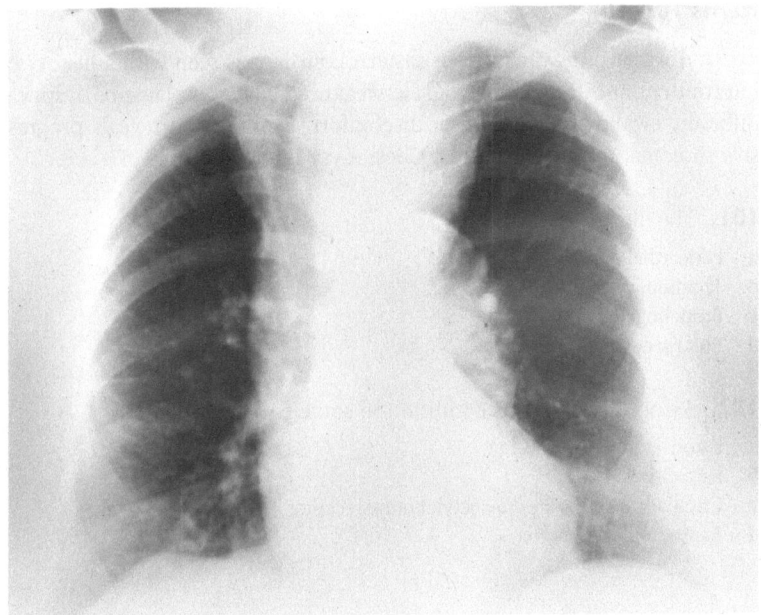

Fig. 56

Items 101–102

A 45-year-old woman from eastern Louisiana is seen with a history of intermittent and fluctuating muscle weakness. She complains of dyspnea, difficulty swallowing, and chest discomfort. Examination reveals progressive proximal muscle weakness. Chest x-ray is shown in Fig. 57.

101. The likely diagnosis is
a. Pericardial cyst
b. Thymoma
c. Bronchogenic cyst
d. Enteric cyst

102. Associated with this condition in some patients is
a. Eaton-Lambert syndrome
b. Hepatitis
c. Circulating antibodies to acetylcholine receptor
d. Aspiration pneumonia

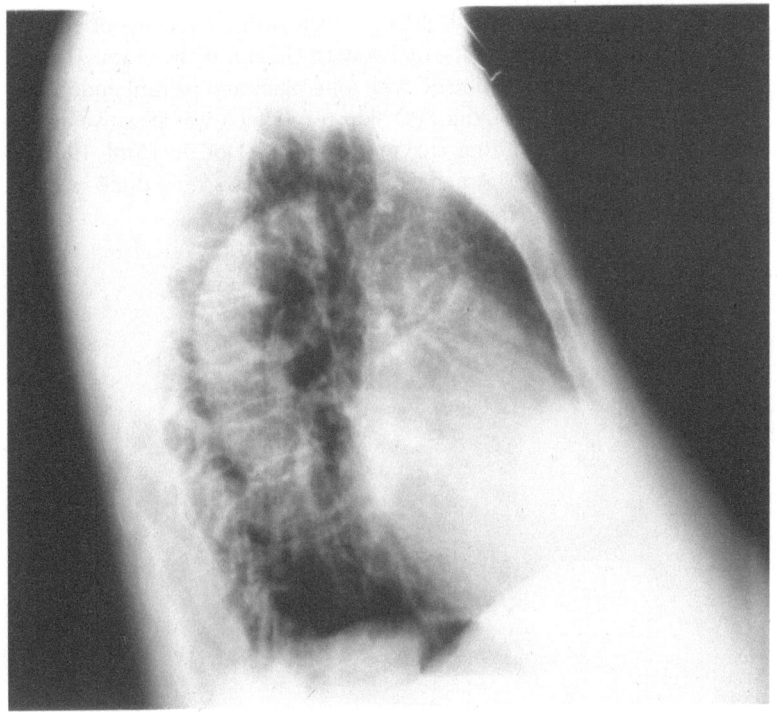

Fig. 57

103. A 38-year-old male truck driver is seen with complaints of chronic cough. He has been living in the midwestern U.S. for many years. About 2 years ago, he had a "flulike illness" with joint pains and painful nodules on the legs. At that time he had a PPD skin test, which was negative, and a serum angiotensin-converting enzyme (ACE) level of 56 U/mL (normal upper limit is 30 U/mL). Among other routine tests now done, a chest x-ray (Fig. 58) is obtained. The most likely diagnosis is

a. Blastomycosis
b. Lymphoma
c. Histoplasmosis
d. Silicosis

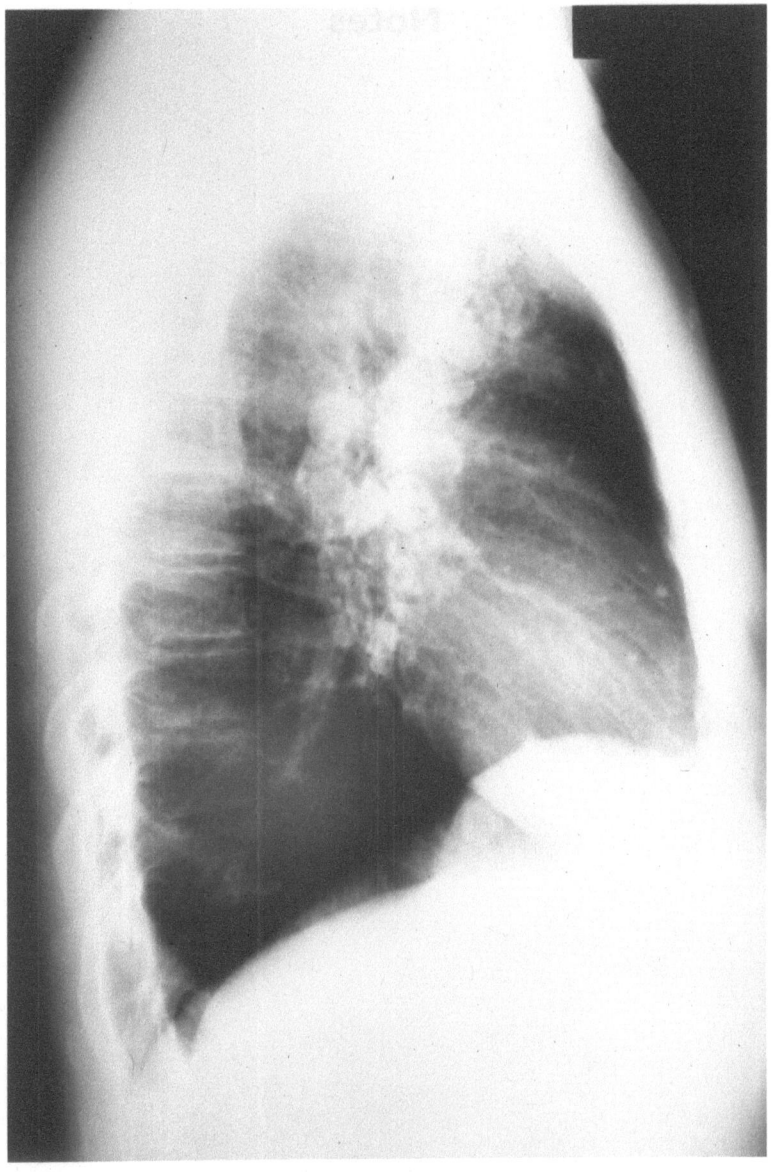

Fig. 58

Notes

Items 104–105

A 30-year-old African American woman presents with decreased exercise tolerance, low-grade fever, fatigue, and cough. She denies any travel or exposure history. On lung exam, she has faint crackles bilaterally. There is no palpable lymphadenopathy. Spirometry is normal except for mild reduction in FEF_{25-75}. PPD is 0 mm. Chest x-rays are shown in Fig. 59.

104. The most likely diagnosis is

a. Sarcoidosis
b. BOOP
c. Hodgkin's lymphoma
d. Hypersensitivity pneumonitis

105. An associated finding with this condition is

a. Clubbing
b. Increased ACE level
c. Increased diffusion on pulmonary function tests
d. Osteoporosis

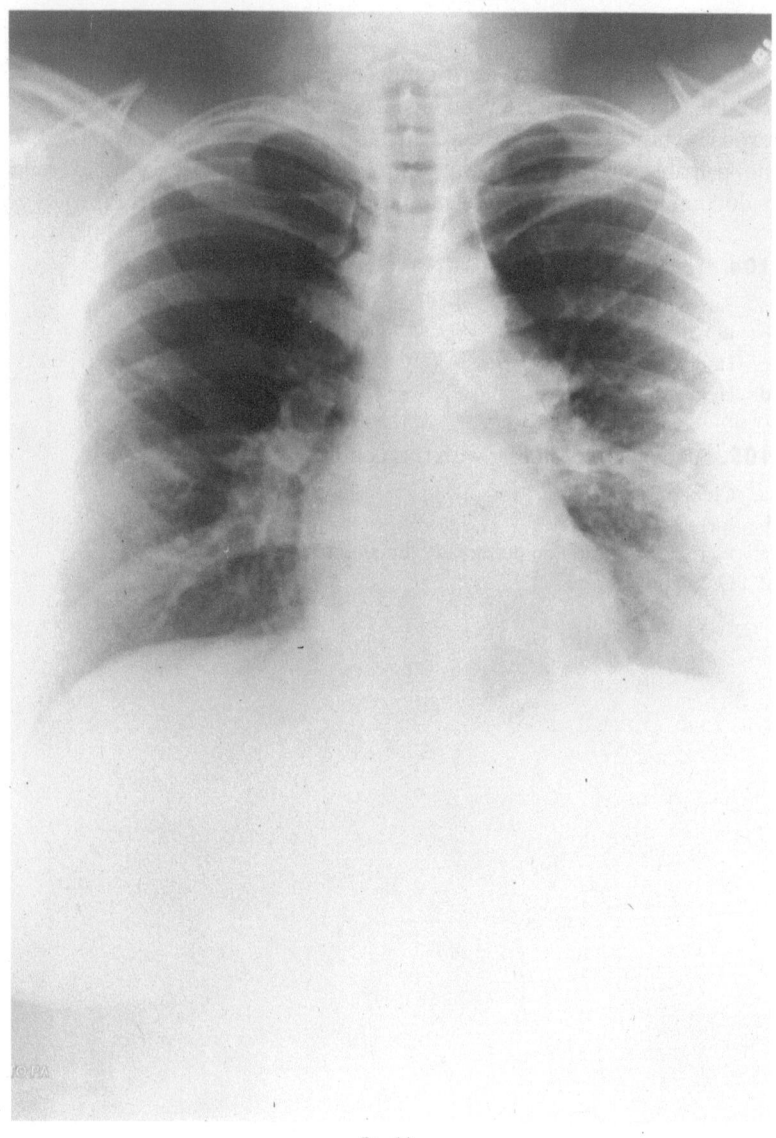

Fig. 59a

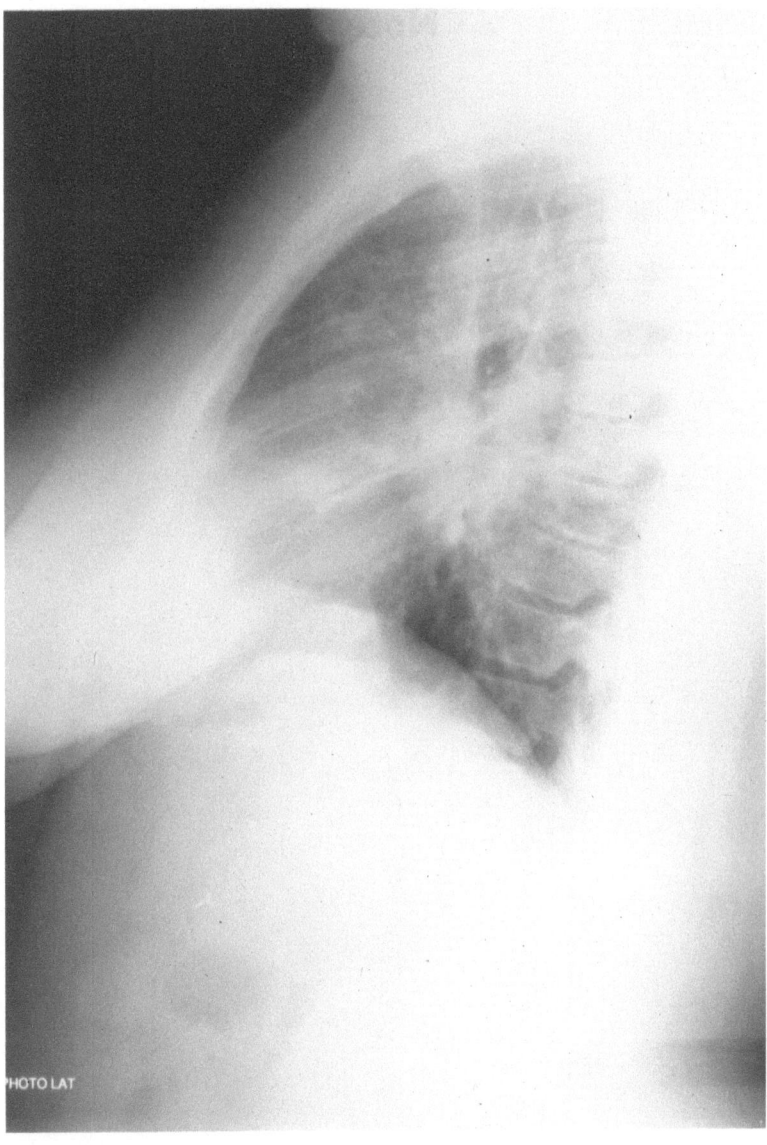

Fig. 59b

Notes

Items 106–107

A 41-year-old male schoolteacher, a nonsmoker, presents with lightheadedness and increased shortness of breath with "lack of stamina" and chest pain. On physical examination, vital signs are normal. The patient is overweight with a BMI of 33. CVS exam reveals a left parasternal heave with a harsh grade 3/6 systolic flow murmur and a loud P_2 sound. Chest radiographs are shown below in Fig. 60.

106. What is the most likely diagnosis?
a. Mitral stenosis
b. Pulmonary hypertension
c. Chronic bronchitis with cor pulmonale
d. Deconditioning due to obesity

107. What is the next management option?
a. Pulmonary function tests
b. Exercise test
c. Echocardiography
d. Pulmonary rehabilitation with an aggressive exercise program

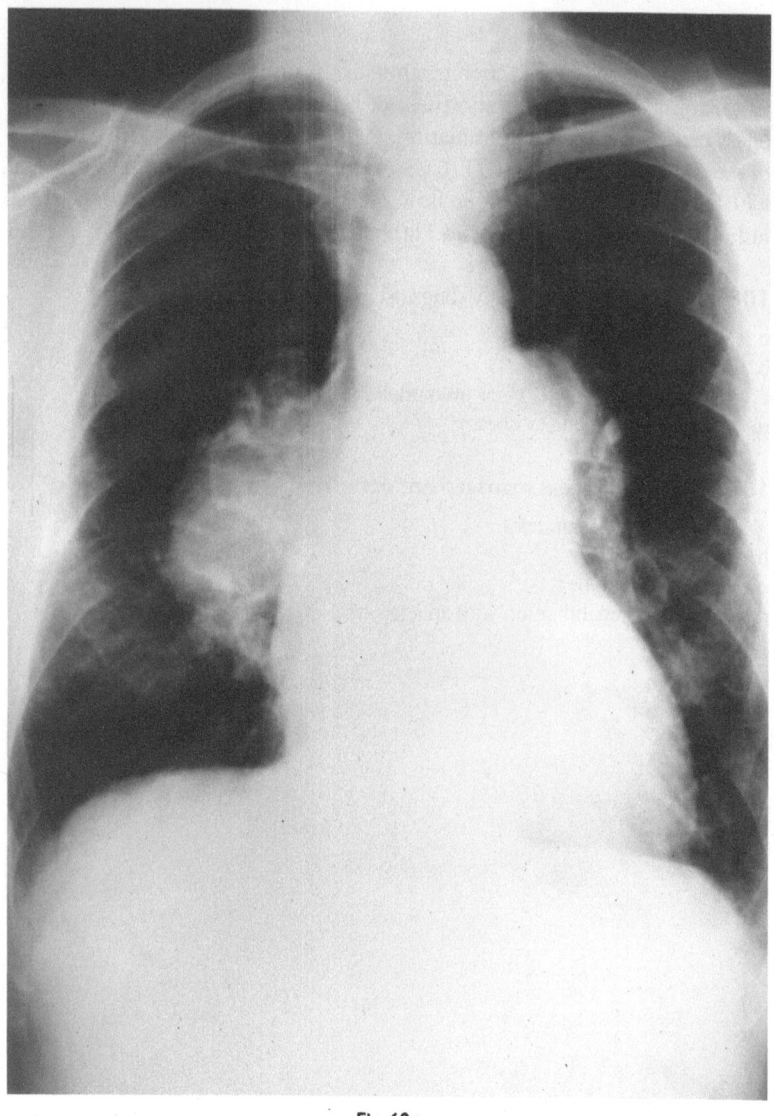

Fig. 60a

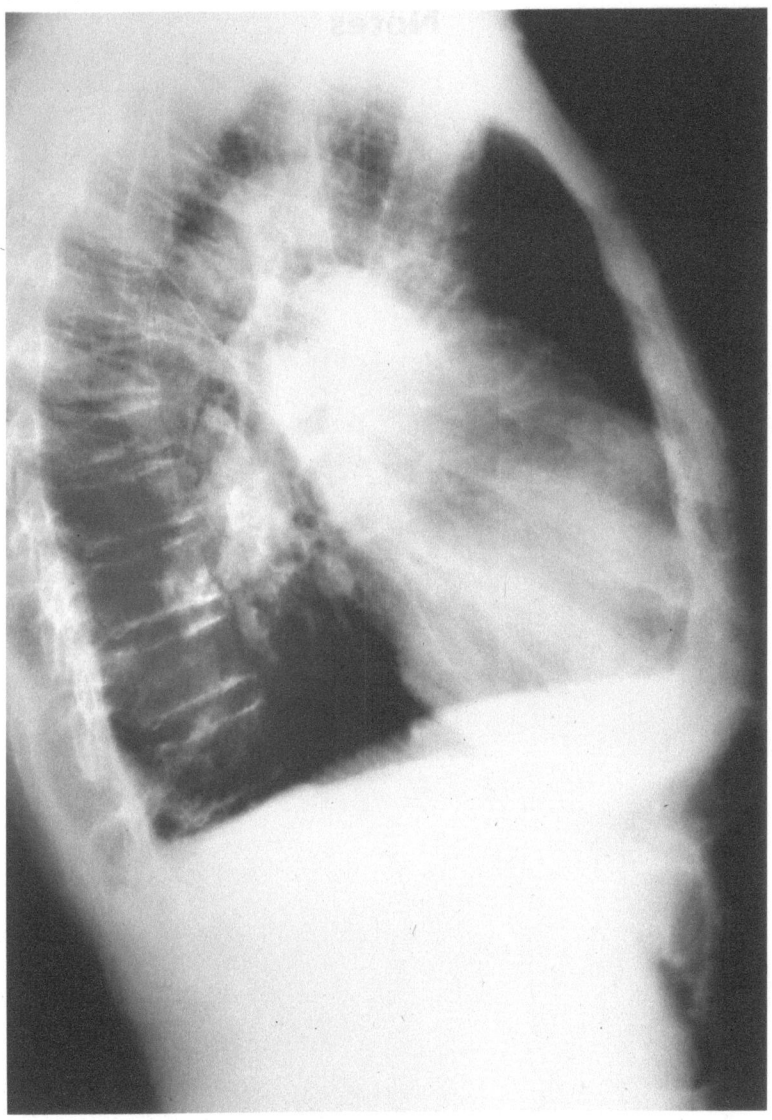

Fig. 60b

Notes

Items 108–109

A 60-year-old woman from Honduras with a history of uncontrolled hypertension is admitted with mild anterior chest pain. She denies any nausea, vomiting, diaphoresis. On physical examination, vital signs are: pulse 100 bpm; temperature normal; respirations 25/min; blood pressure 200/120 mm Hg. On general exam, the patient appears anxious and agitated. Pertinent findings include: heart exam—normal sinus rhythm, with soft systolic murmur, loud A_2; funduscopy—severe exudates and hemorrhages. Laboratory data: Hb 11 g/dL; Hct 33%; WBCs 11.5/μL; BUN 40 mg/dL; creatinine 1.3 mg/dL; sodium 129 mEq/L; potassium 4.5 mEq/L. Cardiac enzymes are normal. EKG shows LVH with strain. Chest radiographs are shown below in Fig. 61.

108. What is the most likely diagnosis?

a. Left ventricular aneurysm
b. Congestive heart failure
c. Neurofibroma
d. Aortic aneurysm

109. While controlling the patient's BP, what is the immediate next diagnostic step?

a. Echocardiogram
b. CT scan
c. Ultrasound of chest
d. Repeat chest x-ray with lordotic view

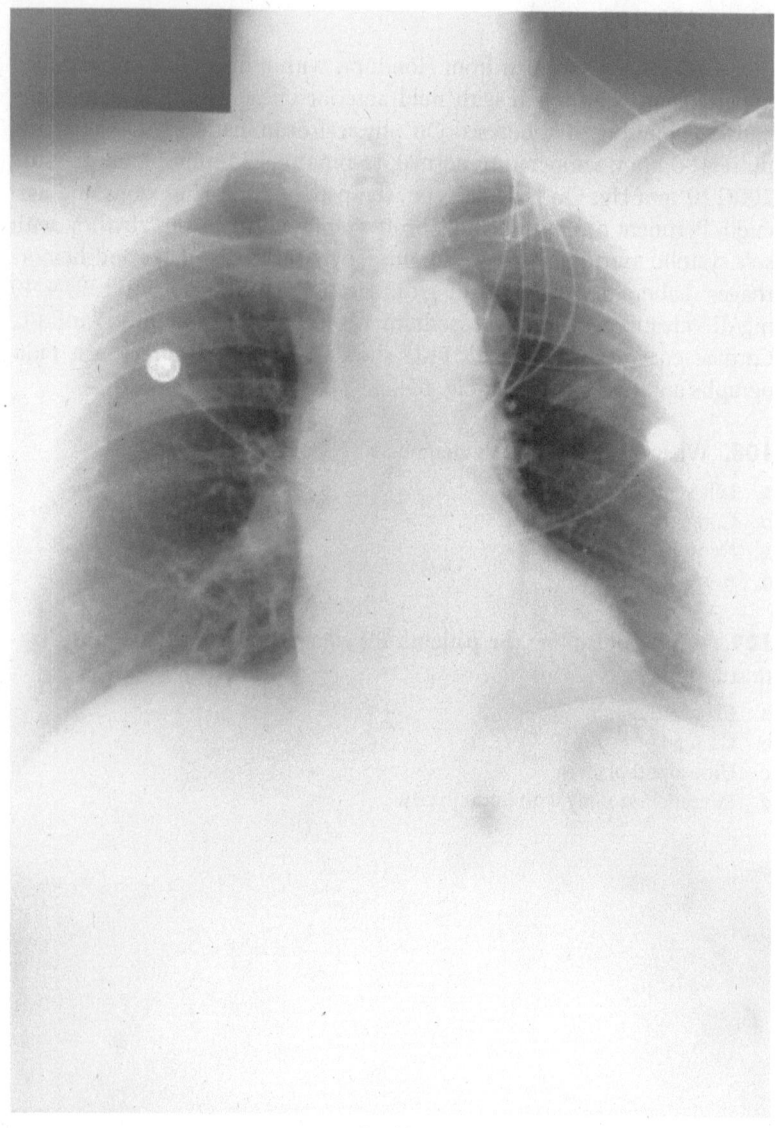

Fig. 61a

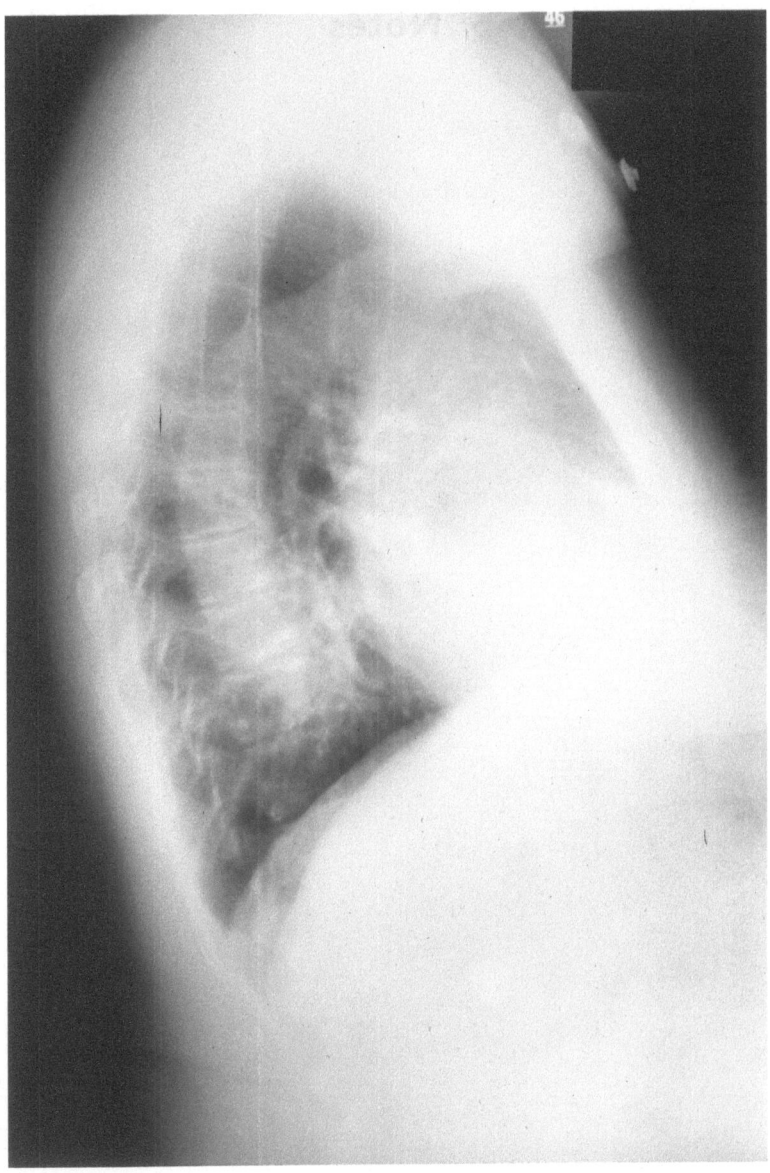

Fig. 61b

Notes

110. A 68-year-old female smoker is admitted with progressive weakness, weight loss, and dysphagia. Physical exam: pulse 110 bpm; temperature normal; respirations 18/min; blood pressure 110/60 mm Hg. The patient appears cachectic on general exam. Laboratory data: Hb 9 g/dL; Hct 27%; BUN 13 mg/dL; creatinine 0.4 mg/dL; sodium 124 mEq/L; potassium 3.8 mEq/L. Chest x-rays are shown in Fig. 62. An associated symptom that may signal mediastinal involvement and inoperability is

a. Cough
b. Clubbing
c. Steady boring chest pain
d. Diaphoresis

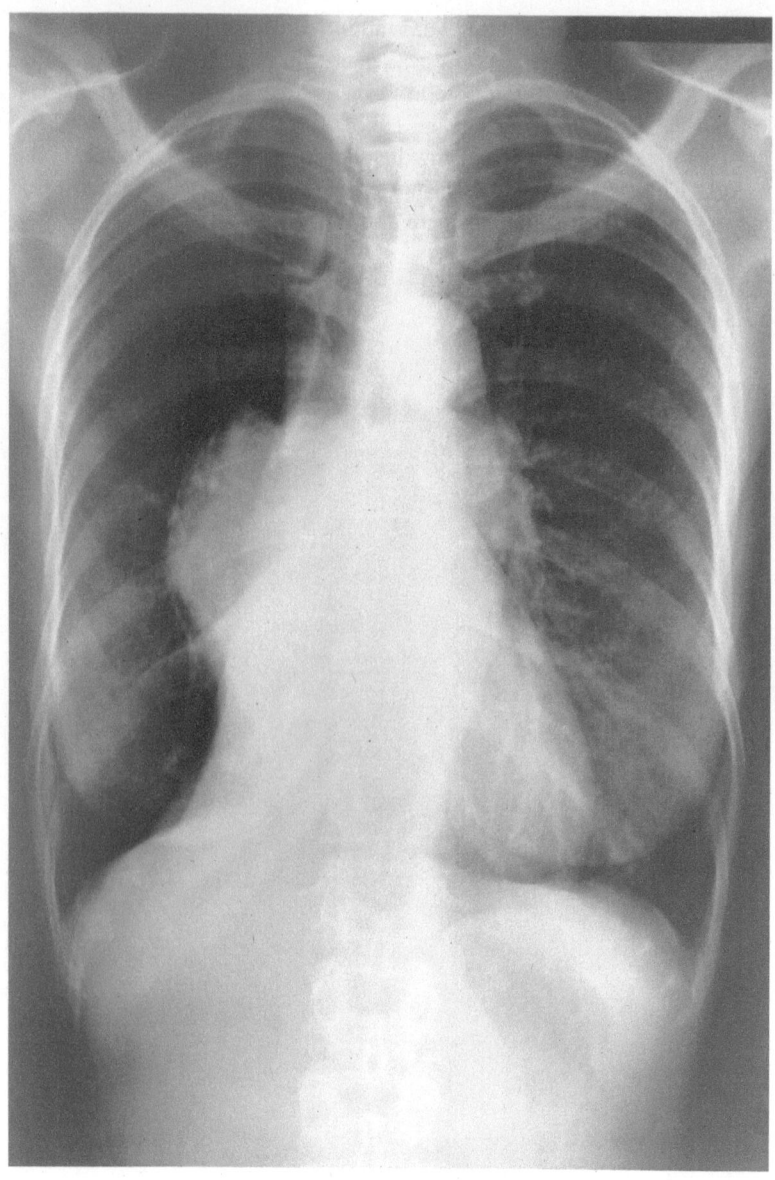

Fig. 62a

Mediastinal Compartments

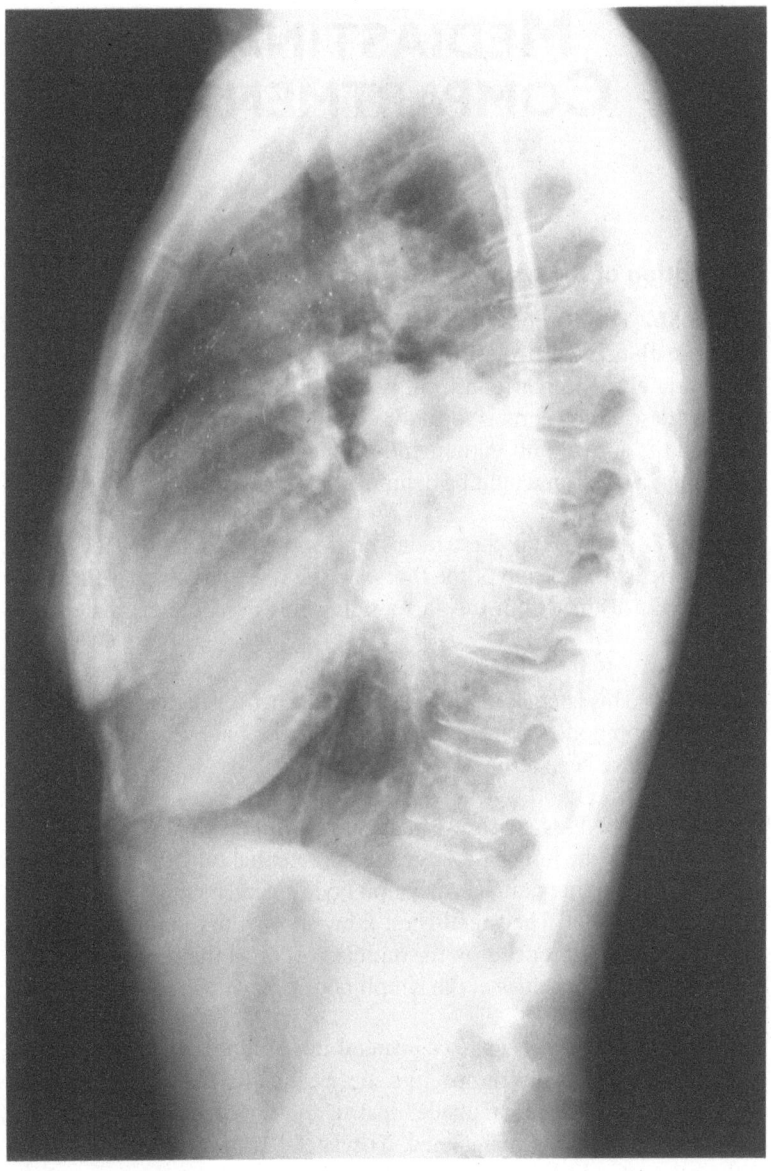

Fig. 62b

MEDIASTINAL COMPARTMENTS

Answers

Description of X-rays in This Chapter

Figure 56. This PA chest film demonstrates a large superior mediastinal shadow with marked right displacement of the trachea. There is minimum thickening of the minor fissure with some small atelectatic streaks on the left. The descending aorta is tortuous and shows a small amount of calcification in the aortic knob. Although this film is most consistent with a thyroid goiter, a CT scan would be definitive.

Figure 57. This lateral chest radiograph shows an anterior mediastinal mass in the lower portion of the thorax in the retrosternal space. It is well defined and distinct from the surrounding soft tissue pericardial/cardiac shadow.

Figure 58. This lateral chest x-ray shows distinct calcified hilar and paratracheal lymph nodes. Some of the calcified nodes have distinct peripheral rims; these have been termed "eggshell" calcifications.

Figure 59. The PA view shows bilateral hilar fullness with increased linear markings in the lung base, suggesting interstitial lung disease. There is a suggestion of right paratracheal lymph node enlargement with no distinct lateral tracheal wall. The lateral chest x-ray shows the rounded lucency of the left upper lobe bronchus in the middle portion of the chest surrounded by the soft tissue opacities of the lymph nodes.

Figure 60. The PA view shows bilateral hilar fullness with well-defined soft tissue opacities. These opacities taper caudally. The aorta is normal, there is no paratracheal lymphadenopathy, and the concavity of the aortopulmonary window is maintained. The lateral shows the hilar shadows with an anterior and posterior prominence in the infraaortic area with no paratracheal fullness. Although a CT with contrast is needed to confirm that these opacities are due to enlarged pulmonary arteries, the shape and contour of the shadows make a vascular shadow the most likely radiographic diagnosis.

Figure 61. The PA view shows normal lung parenchyma with no acute or active process. The cardiac size and pulmonary vasculature appear normal. The descending aortic shadow appears more prominent and there is a double density around the aortic arch. On the lateral, there is some haziness in the retrosternal space and a bulge is seen in the superior aspect of the aortic arch shadow. The ascending aorta appears to have calcification in the anterior wall. These findings are consistent with an aortic arch aneurysm.

Figure 62. The PA view shows a large, well-defined opacity in the right hilum. The ascending aorta shadow is not silhouetted, suggesting that this is a posterior opacity. The left hilum and the left PA appear normal. The lateral confirms the posterior mediastinal location of the opacity. Here it appears more irregular and is distinctly posterior to where the right pulmonary artery shadow would be on the lateral. This picture is consistent with a posterior mediastinal mass, possibly an esophageal tumor.

General Discussion

Anatomically, the mediastinum is divided into four compartments. Although essentially arbitrary, this division helps in narrowing down the radiological differential diagnosis. Some radiologists have used the margin of the aortic arch to divide this area into superior and inferior or supra- and infravascular mediastinal compartments. However, the compartmental demarcations are best outlined on a lateral chest radiograph. The anatomic landmarks and divisions are:

- *Superior mediastinum:* above the level of the aortic arch shadow. It is difficult to evaluate due to superimposed soft tissue and bony shadows.
- *Anterior mediastinum:* the retrosternal airspace with the posterior border running anterior to the great vessels, alongside the ascending aorta and anterior and superior to the heart.
- *Middle mediastinum:* encompasses a space that runs from the posterior border of the esophagus to the level of the hilum and then inferiorly along the posterior margin of the heart.

- *Posterior mediastinum:* posterior to the posterior margin of the heart and extending to the posterior thorax.

The common anterior mediastinal masses are the so-called **6 Ts:** thymoma, teratoma, thyroid, thoracic aorta, trauma, "terrible lymphoma." Superior mediastinal masses include substernal thyroid goiters and vascular aneurysmal lesions along with neoplastic and lymph node lesions. Esophageal lesions are sometimes overlooked when evaluating a superior mediastinal mass. The middle mediastinal masses are related to lymph nodes, pulmonary vasculature, or pericardial and cardiac disease. The hilum forms the root of the middle mediastinal structures; bilateral hilar lymphadenopathy (BHL) or pulmonary artery lesions are seen in this area. The causes of BHL will be discussed later in this section. The pericardial and cardiac lesions will be discussed in Chap. 15. Posterior mediastinal masses are related to the posterior structures such as the esophagus in the lower portion and the aorta. Paraspinous pathology and neurogenic tumors are also seen in this region.

Specific Discussion

98–100. The answers are 98-a, 99-c, 100-d. The question concerns primarily the chest radiograph abnormality, which is an incidental finding in this elderly patient with urosepsis. The CXR is consistent with substernal goiter. These are usually benign, and only infrequently large enough to significantly compress the upper airway. However, the extent of tracheal deviation in this patient requires further evaluation via CT scan. A flow volume loop would be helpful to rule out extrathoracic obstruction and potential for stridor and respiratory distress. The clinical feature and the bilateral smooth contour of the opacity make the other options less likely.

101–102. The answers are 101-b, 102-c. The patient has an anterior mediastinal mass, which is a thymoma. Thymoma usually occurs at the level of or just superior to the hilum. There are four well-established paraneoplastic or clinical syndromes associated with thymoma. (1) Bronchiectasis results from repeated infections from acquired hypoglobulinemia occurring in 10% of patients with thymoma. (2) Primary red cell aplasia occurs in 5% of the patients with thymoma with normocytic, normochromic anemia. Of all patients with primary red cell aplasia, 50% will have accompanying thymoma. Thymectomy will induce remission. (3) Myasthenia gravis resulting in muscle weakness is due to antibodies directed at the postsynaptic acetylcholine receptors. Up to 40% of patients with thymoma have myasthenia gravis, but thymectomy rarely alters the clinical course. (4) Extrathymic malignancies, lymphoma, thyroid cancer, and lung cancer occur in 20% of thymoma patients. Eaton-Lambert syndrome is a rare paraneoplastic neuromuscular defect in which the autoantibodies are directed against P/Q-type voltage-gated calcium channels called VGCCs. The presence of autoantibodies blocks calcium influx into the nerves. It is associated with certain malignancies, especially small cell lung cancer. The Tensilon test is not always definitive in patients with mysasthenia gravis; assessment for antibodies to acetylcholine receptors, detected in 90% of patients with myasthenia gravis, is the test of choice. Hepatitis and aspiration pneumonia are not associated with thymoma.

103. The answer is c. The patient is from an endemic area where histoplasmosis is prevalent. The clinical symptoms with erythema nodosum are consistent with this diagnosis. Serum ACE level is typically increased in sarcoidosis but can also be increased in histoplasmosis. The chest x-ray showing "eggshell" calcifications is seen in granulomatous diseases, sarcoidosis, and silicosis. As there is no history of exposure to silica or silica-related occupational hazard, option c is the best answer.

104–105. The answers are 104-a, 105-b. Bilateral hilar lymphadenopathy (BHL) in a young African American female with non-specific symptoms is suggestive of sarcoidosis. Generally the other causes of BHL include granulomatous diseases, carcinomatosis, and lymphomatosis. Bronchiolitis obliterans (BO) is defined pathologically as injury to small airways with granulation tissue reaction and repair resulting in obliterative bronchiolar scarring. When this process extends into the alveolar ducts, it is termed organizing pneumonia and the entity is called bronchiolitis obliterans with organizing pneumonia (BOOP). It is usually secondary to a prolonged viral or infectious illness, inhalational or toxic exposure, chronic antigenic insult, or connective tissue disorders such as rheumatoid arthritis and presents with persistent infiltrates on a chest x-ray. It can lead to pulmonary fibrosis. The clinical scenario and CXR are not consistent with this diagnosis in this patient. Hypersensitivity pneumonitis is generally secondary to an inhalational exposure causing pulmonary infiltrates. Sarcoidosis is not associated with clubbing or osteoporosis. It causes bone cyst formations and deformities and leads to reduced diffusing capacity on pulmonary function tests.

106–107. The answers are 106-b, 107-c. The symptoms described in this patient and the characteristic CXR are consistent with pulmonary hypertension. This could be further worked up and confirmed by an echocardiogram to estimate PA pressures. Chronic bronchitis is unlikely in this nonsmoker, and deconditioning would not give the physical signs observed. There is no clinical or radiographic evidence of mitral stenosis. PFT and exercise test would be abnormal but nonspecific, and aggressive exercise programs would be contraindicated.

108–109. The answers are 108-d, 109-a. Chest symptoms in an uncontrolled hypertensive with end organ damage are suggestive of either an acute coronary event or aortic dissection. The ECG does not show any acute ischemia or injury pattern. CXR reveals a double shadow in the region of the aortic arch, suggesting a dissection of undetermined age and/or an aneurysm. An ultrasound of the chest would be unhelpful; repeat chest x-ray would be redundant and the lordotic view is only helpful for evaluating apical pulmonary disease. A renal scan would probably only confirm the renal insufficiency as depicted by the increased creatinine. A CT scan would be most helpful to confirm this diagnosis, but has some risk in a patient with azotemia.

110. The answer is c. This large posterior mediastinal mass is an esophageal lesion, and the presence of steady, constant, boring pain is indicative of mediastinal involvement and therefore inoperability. Cough may be due to aspiration or laryngeal reflux; clubbing can at times be seen in both benign and malignant lesions of the esophagus and does not indicate mediastinal involvement or inoperability.

CARDIAC AND PERICARDIAL DISEASE

DIRECTIONS: Each item below contains a question or incomplete statement followed by suggested responses. Select the **one best** response to each question.

Items 111–112

A 47-year-old woman is seen with a 1-wk history of progressive shortness of breath, increasing pedal edema, weight loss, and low-grade fever. She has a 40-pack-year smoking history. Physical examination: pulse 138 bpm; respirations 34/min; blood pressure 100/88 mm Hg with pulsus paradoxus of 22 mm. Pertinent findings: increased jugular venous distension, normal sinus rhythm with distant heart sounds, and an apex beat that is difficult to palpate. Chest x-ray is shown below in Fig. 63.

111. What is the most likely diagnosis?
a. Cardiac tamponade
b. Cardiomyopathy
c. Pericardial effusion without tamponade
d. Cor pulmonale

112. Another finding associated with this diagnosis would be
a. Kussmaul sign
b. Low voltage on ECG
c. Left ventricular hypertrophy
d. Pulmonary edema

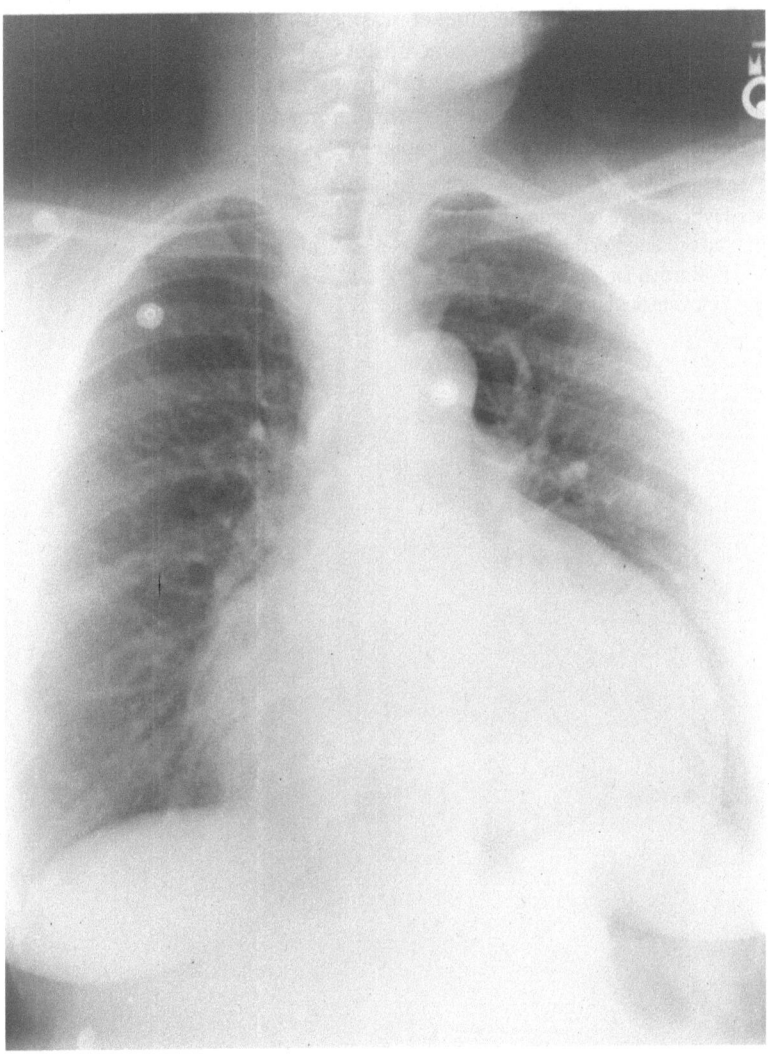

Fig. 63

113. A 67-year-old male smoker was seen in the ER for evaluation of cough and treated for acute bronchitis. A CXR done at that time prompted a referral to the chest clinic. The patient gives a past history of myocardial infarction, but at the moment is asymptomatic. BP is 128/80 and cardiopulmonary exam is unremarkable. PPD is 7 mm. CXR is shown in Fig. 64. The likely diagnosis is

a. Hypertensive cardiomyopathy
b. Tuberculous pericarditis
c. Epicardial fat pad
d. Left ventricular aneurysm

Cardiac and Pericardial Disease 223

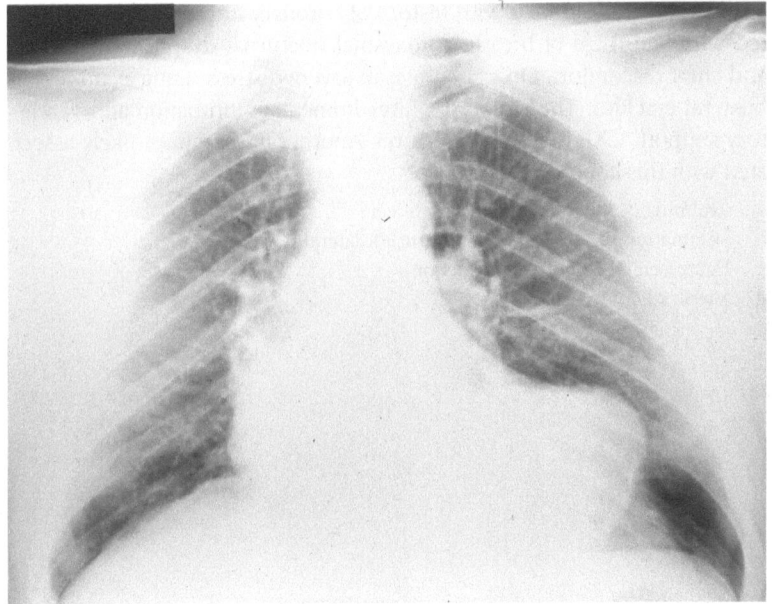

Fig. 64

114. A 46-year-old man with history of coronary artery disease is admitted with shortness of breath, paroxysmal nocturnal dyspnea, orthopnea, and chest discomfort. On exam, he is in severe distress. Lung exam reveals bilateral crackles. The patient requires immediate intubation and ventilatory support. CXR is shown in Fig. 65. Another finding most likely associated with this condition is

a. Clubbing of the left hand and both feet
b. Summation gallop heard best in the left lateral position
c. Decreased DLCO on lung function
d. Massive hemoptysis

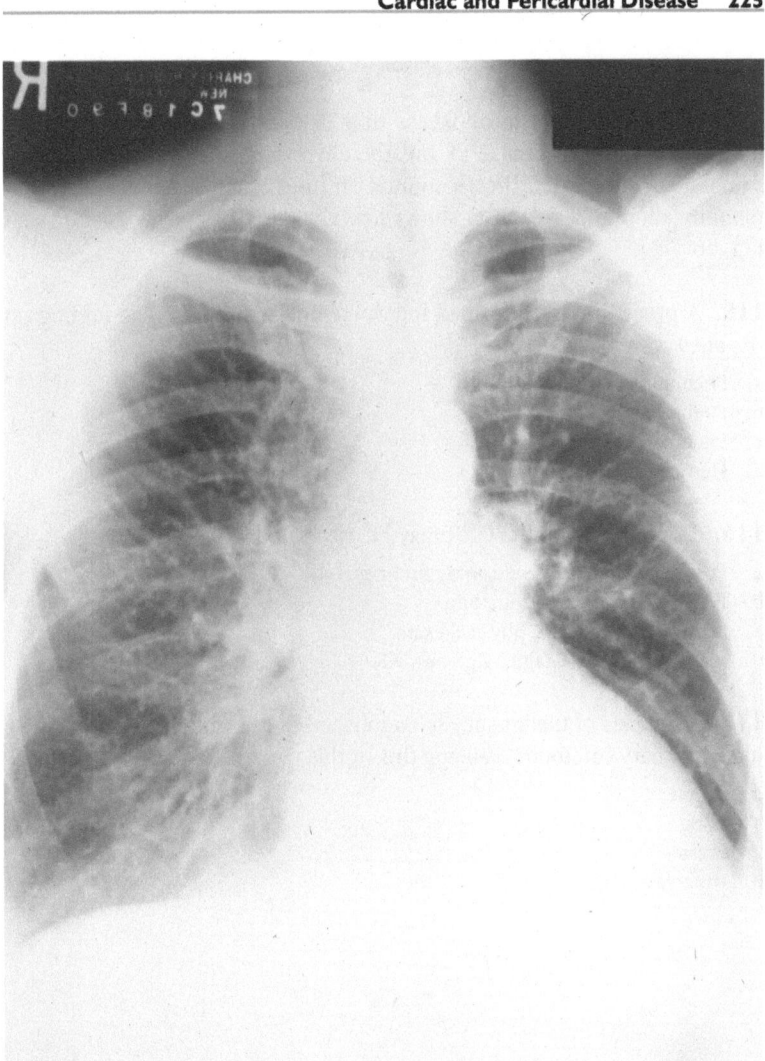

Fig. 65

Items 115–117

A 42-year-old female smoker with a 20-pack-year history is admitted with progressive shortness of breath. On exam, she has distant heart sounds with decreased breath sounds on lung exam bilaterally. No summation gallop is heard. ECG shows low voltage. Chest x-ray is shown in Fig. 66.

115. A procedure is performed for worsening symptoms. The finding on the chest x-ray is

a. Pneumomediastinum
b. Pneumopericardium
c. Pneumothorax
d. Herniation of the right lung

116. The findings on the CXR may be associated with

a. Positional change of chest x-ray findings
b. Pericardial rub on auscultation
c. Hamman's crunch on physical exam
d. "Continuous diaphragm" sign on CXR

117. Diagnosis of malignancy is established by the above procedure. The likely primary carcinoma causing this in this patient is

a. Colon
b. Lung
c. Breast
d. Pancreas

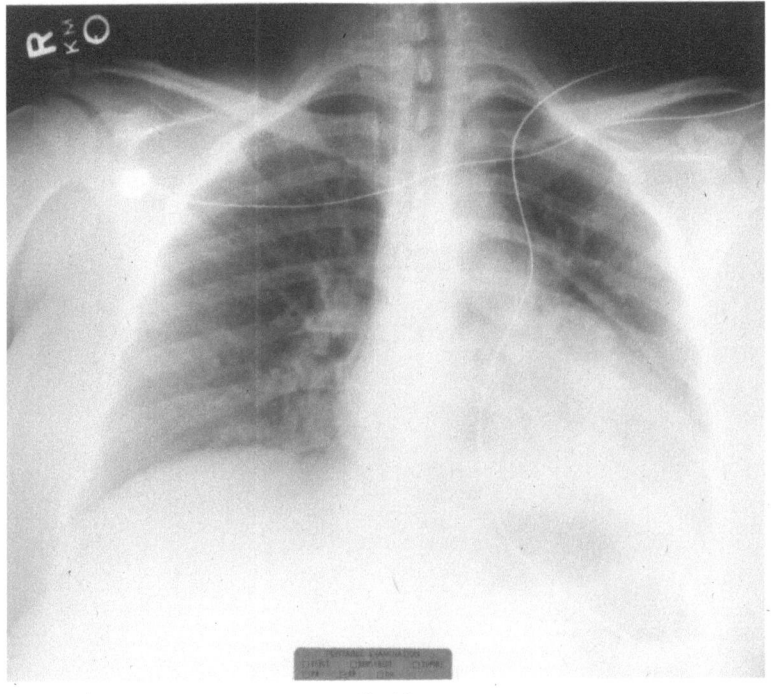

Fig. 66

Notes

Items 118-119

A 59-year-old Vietnamese-American female nonsmoker with a history of hypertension is seen for upper respiratory symptoms and cough. Chest x-rays are done (Fig. 67) and the patient is treated symptomatically. When it is pointed out to her that her chest x-ray is abnormal, she says she has had pleurisy in the past and brings in an old chest x-ray taken at the time of her immigration to the U.S. 5 years ago. That x-ray is essentially the same as the current one.

118. The CXR shown is consistent with a diagnosis of

a. Tuberculosis
b. Chronic pleural effusion
c. Asbestosis
d. Old trauma

119. This patient is most likely to develop

a. Kussmaul sign
b. Obstructive dysfunction on PFTs
c. Lung cancer
d. Hemoptysis

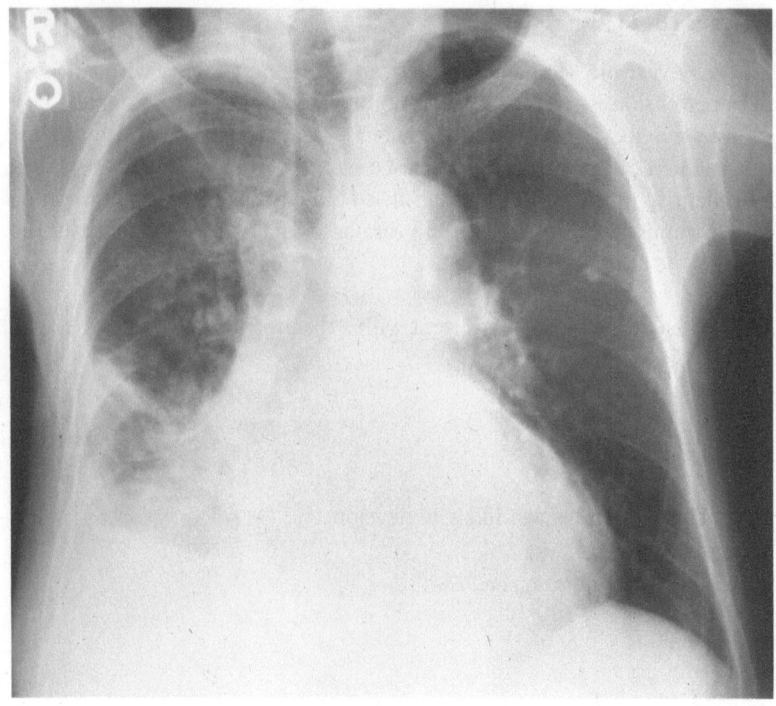

Fig. 67a

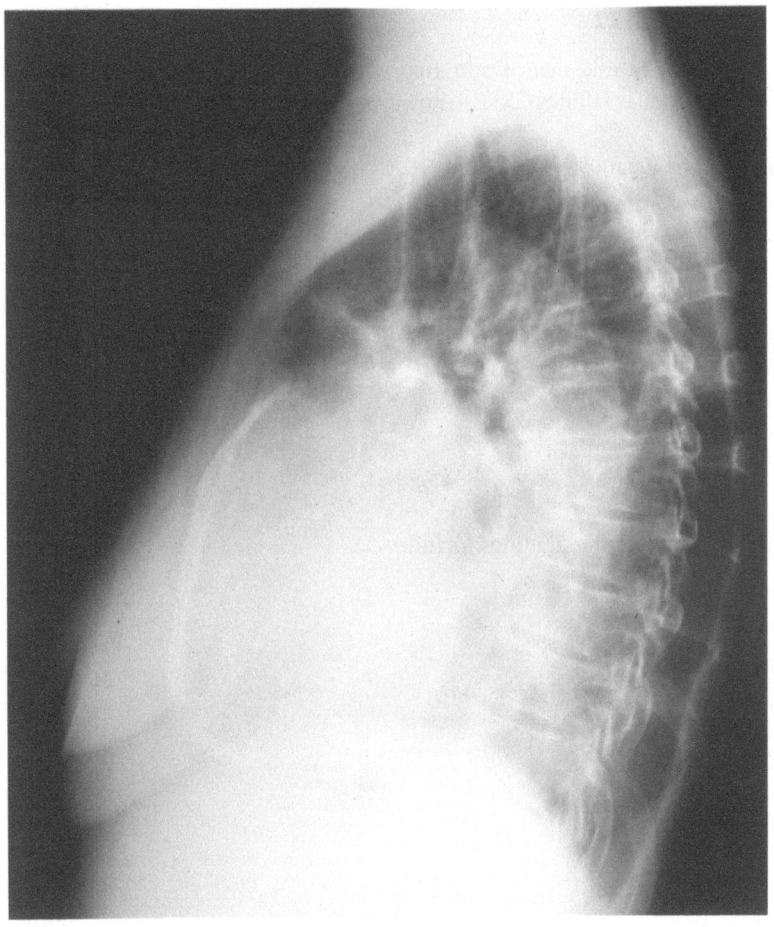

Fig. 67b

Items 120–122

A 48-year-old man is admitted with shortness of breath and signs of left ventricular failure. CXR is shown in Fig. 68.

120. The diagnosis based on the CXR is associated with
a. A diastolic rumble
b. Soft first heart sound
c. Clubbing
d. Koilonychia

121. Complications of this condition include all except
a. Hemoptysis
b. Endocarditis
c. Atrial flutter/fibrillation
d. Atrial myxoma

122. Radiographic findings include
a. Cavitary disease
b. Pneumothorax
c. Widened carinal angle
d. Hilar mass

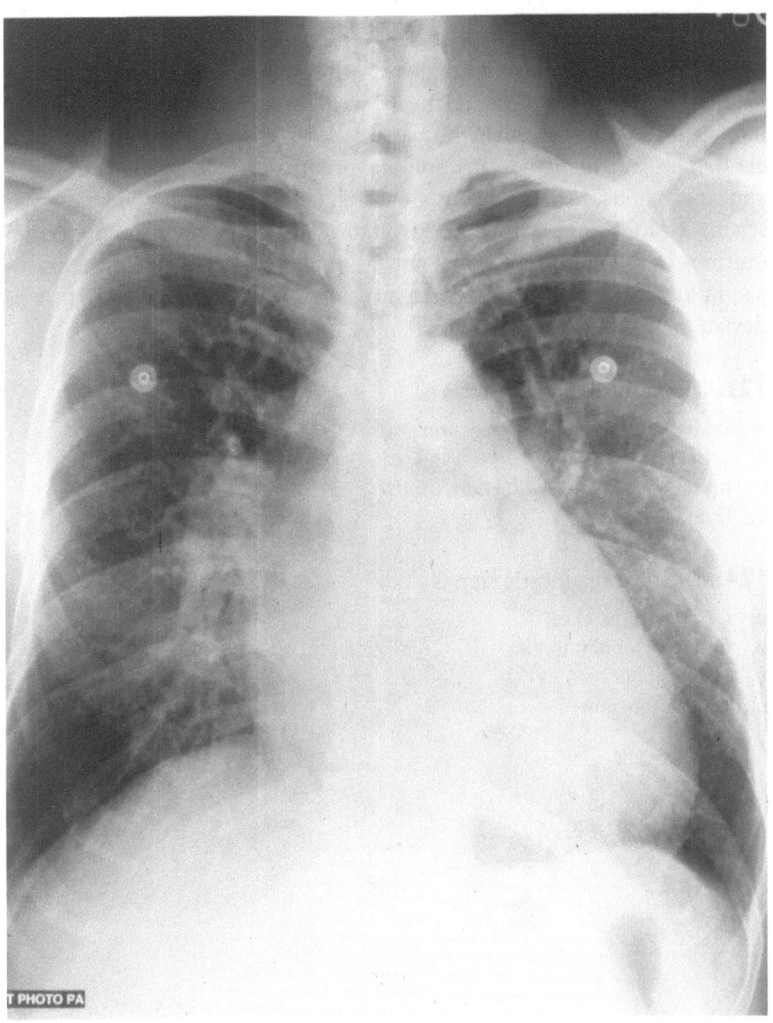

Fig. 68

Items 123-124

A 27-year-old woman is admitted with cough, shortness of breath, and palpitations. She has been relatively well for most of her life, but her mother gives a history that the patient had recurrent "pneumonia" as a child. The patient denies any sputum production. On examination, she appears anxious. Her neck veins are distended and she has a widened split second heart sound with little respiratory variation. A systolic ejection murmur in the pulmonic area is noted. Lung exam reveals bilateral crackles; mild ascites and pedal edema are also noted. EKG shows right axis deviation. CXR is shown in Fig. 69.

123. The most likely diagnosis is
a. Primary pulmonary hypertension
b. Atrial septal defect
c. Immune deficiency with endocarditis
d. Bronchiectasis sicca

124. The next diagnostic step is
a. CT scan of the chest
b. Immunoglobulin levels
c. PPD testing
d. Echocardiogram

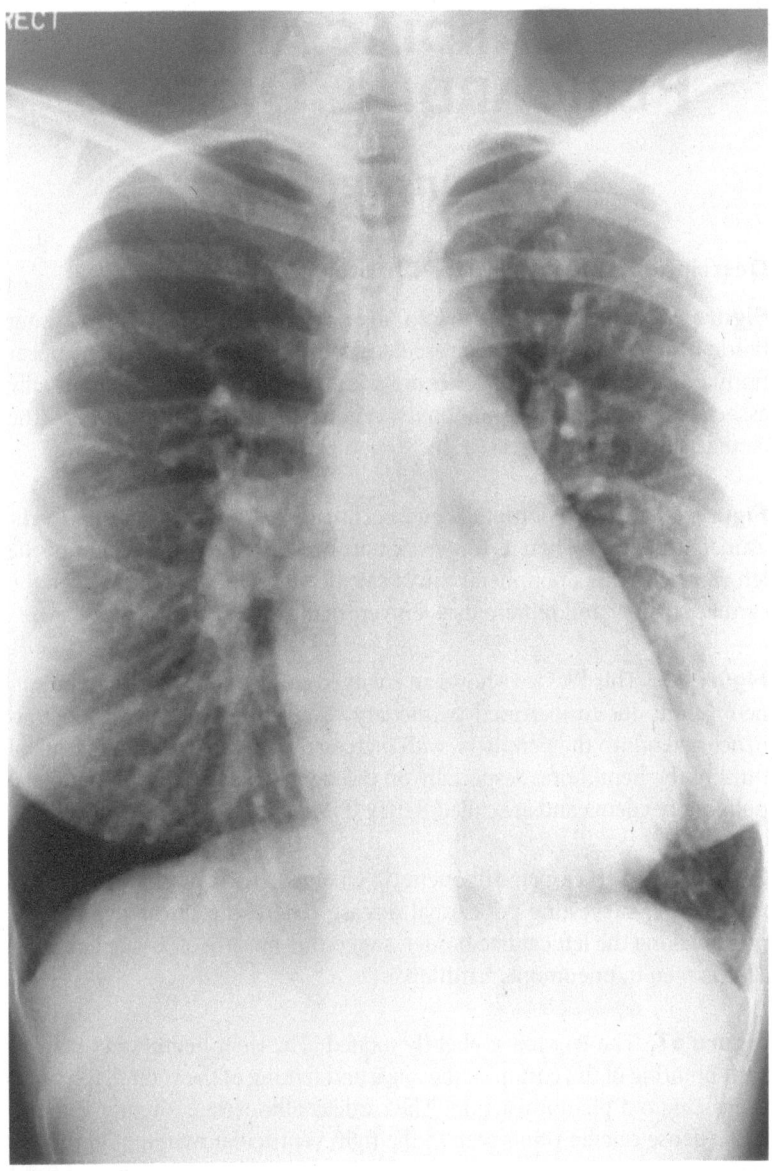

Fig. 69

CARDIAC AND PERICARDIAL DISEASE

Answers

Description of X-rays in This Chapter

Figure 63. This PA view shows a large cardiac silhouette with a "water bottle heart." The pulmonary vasculature and the vascular pedicle appear normal. Large cardiac silhouettes are seen in cardiomegaly and are usually associated with signs of pulmonary venous congestion. In this case, the cardiac silhouette is increased due to pericardial effusion.

Figure 64. This AP lordotic view accentuates middle and anterior mediastinal structures. There is a convex outward opacity in the region of the left ventricle with a peripheral rim of calcification. It is contiguous with the cardiac shadow and represents a left ventricular aneurysm.

Figure 65. This PA view shows an enlarged cardiac silhouette with prominent hilum due to increased pulmonary vasculature. The vascular prominence extends to the periphery, with increased transverse lines in the lateral third of the hemithorax, especially on the right. These represent interstitial pulmonary edema and are called Kerley B lines.

Figure 66. The cardiac silhouette is enlarged, with normal pulmonary vasculature, suggesting pericardial disease. There is a linear hyperlucent margin along the left cardiac border, suggesting an air–soft tissue interface. This is seen in pneumopericardium.

Figure 67. The PA view is slightly rotated. The right hemithorax is small with blunting of the costophrenic angle and tenting of the right diaphragm, suggesting old pleural reaction. The cardiac silhouette is slightly globular and a dense calcific rim is seen in the right ventricular margin. On the lateral this dense calcification can be seen in a circumferential manner around the cardiac shadow. This is indicative of pericardial calcification.

Figure 68. The cardiac silhouette is large, with prominent pulmonary vasculature and increased vascular markings in the lower and lateral portions of the hemithorax. Transverse lines can be seen in the lateral one-third of the lower right lung zone. These are Kerley B lines and are indicative of interstitial pulmonary edema. There is straightening of the left heart border from the aortic shadow, called *mitralization* of the heart. The carinal angle appears to be about 90° which is wider than normal, also suggesting an enlarged subcarinal left atrial appendage. This chest x-ray is consistent with pulmonary edema and left atrial and left ventricular enlargement.

Figure 69. The cardiac silhouette is normal in size, but the pulmonary vasculature is prominent and the AP window is full. The interlobar branches appear large. There is pulmonary plethora with increased vasculature, especially in the right lower zone and the left upper zone, with increase in size of the arterial shadows suggesting increased pulmonary blood flow.

General Discussion

Kerley A lines are a coarse network of linear strands about 2 to 6 cm long and 1 mm thick within the lung substance in the central zone midway between the axillary lung margin and the heart. The orientation of these lines does not conform to the distribution of the bronchovascular bundles; they represent edema of the central pulmonary septa and perilymphatic connective tissue. They extend medially to the hilum. They are seen in pneumoconiosis, lymphangitic carcinoma, and pulmonary edema (in which case they may be reversible).

Kerley B lines represent edema of the interlobular septa and are approximately 1 cm in length and oriented in the horizontal plane perpendicular to the axillary pleura. They are best seen just above the costophrenic angle and are reversible and transient in pulmonary edema. They may be permanent and irreversible in chronic pulmonary venous hypertension, pneumoconiosis, sarcoidosis, and lymphangitic carcinoma.

Kerley C lines are another manifestation of septal edema and are actually Kerley B lines in the midzone seen en face.

Specific Discussion

111-112. The answers are 111-a, 112-b. The presence of pulsus paradoxus with distant heart sounds suggests cardiac tamponade secondary to pericardial effusion as seen on the chest x-ray. The associated finding would be a low voltage on ECG due to an effusion. Pulsus alternans may also be seen. The Kussmaul sign is seen with constrictive pericarditis. Left ventricular hypertrophy and pulmonary edema suggest left ventricular failure. This is not necessarily associated with cardiac tamponade and pericardial disease.

113. The answer is d. Left ventricular aneurysm is usually secondary to myocardial infarction and may calcify. A true aneurysmal dilatation occurs anterolaterally and may require elective surgery. False aneurysms occur posteriorly and usually signify a contained rupture, which requires emergent surgical resection. In this case, the chest x-ray and the history of previous myocardial infarction make option d the best answer.

114. The answer is b. The clinical history is consistent with left ventricular failure secondary to an acute coronary event. One of the signs of heart failure is a summation gallop. The chest x-ray is consistent with this diagnosis also. Diffusion is increased in congestive heart failure due to decreased transit time at the alveolar capillary interface; hemoptysis is generally mild with pink frothy sputum, and clubbing is not present.

115–117. The answers are 115-b, 116-a, 117-b. The chest x-ray shows a pneumopericardium. This refers to the presence of air within the pericardial sac. Pathologically, air can enter the pericardium from the mediastinum near the pulmonary veins. Air can also develop within the pericardium due to production by gas-forming organisms in cases of infection. At times the pneumopericardium may be complicated by the presence of fluid (hydropneumopericardium) or pus (pyopneumopericardium). Closed chest injury with or without perforation of the pericardium is the most frequent nonsurgical cause associated with this kind of pattern. Contiguous organ involvement (pulmonary abscess, bronchogenic carcinoma, esophagitis, perforated gastric ulcer, foreign body) also can result in the involvement of the pericardium and hence cause pneumopericardium. Septicemia causing direct seeding of the pericardial space can also produce a common communication with the lung. With pneumopericardium, the lucent halo of air partially or completely surrounds the heart but does not extend superiorly to the attachments of the pericardium, and the concomitant subcutaneous emphysema is absent. If supine and erect radiographs are obtained, pericardial air will immediately shift in location whereas mediastinal air change will not occur.

The "continuous diaphragm sign" is seen in pneumomediastinum. In this sign, the right and the left hemidiaphragms appear continuous due to mediastinal air present along the diaphragm and below the heart, giving the appearance of a single continuous diaphragm. Both adults and children can develop life-threatening cardiac tamponade due to pneumopericardium. A pericardial rub is a sign of pericarditis and is usually not heard once an effusion develops. The Hamman sign is a crunching noise heard with the apex beat and heard best in the left lateral decubitus position. It is seen in 50% of cases of mediastinal emphysema (pneumomediastinum) and is associated with subcutaneous emphysema in the suprasternal notch. Malignant pericardial effusions are most commonly seen secondary to breast and lung cancer, but local spread is commonly due to the latter.

118–119. The answers are 118-a, 119-a. The chest x-ray shows calcified pericardium. Asbestosis is defined as respiratory impairment with interstitial lung disease. Asbestos exposure causes pleural plaques. This is not seen on the chest x-ray. Tuberculous pericarditis is an unusual manifestation of tuberculosis in much of the Western world. Pericardial involvement occurs in 1% to 4% of all patients with tuberculosis. Tuberculosis is also frequently implicated as a cause of constrictive pericarditis, and the Kussmaul sign is seen in this disorder. In the United States, tuberculosis accounts for about one-fifth of cases of chronic constrictive pericarditis. Tuberculosis accounts for 93% of cases of pericardial effusion in patients coinfected with HIV. There are four stages in the evolution of tuberculous pericarditis. Initially there is a fibrous stage in which the diffused deposits of fibrin develop together with granulomatous reaction. The second stage is effusion within the pericardial sac, believed to be due to a hypersensitivity reaction to tuberculosis protein. The pericardium itself becomes thickened with fibrous exudates. As the effusion resolves, pericardial thickening may develop. With parietal pericardial thickening, myocardial constriction can occur. There is no free pleural fluid. Unilateral pleural reaction may cause restrictive impairment of pulmonary function.

120–122. The answers are 120-a, 121-d, 122-c. The CXR shows acute pulmonary edema with cardiomegaly. Bilateral airspace densities are noted. Pulmonary edema is the result of increased pulmonary venous pressures, i.e., hydrostatic edema, which can be due to volume overload or congestive heart failure. This is usually associated with cardiomegaly, although the heart size may be normal in acute myocardial infarction or acute valvular dysfunction. Impaired pulmonary venous return due to left ventricular failure or mitral valve disease leads to increased pulmonary blood volume. Signs of cephalization of blood flow suggest enlargement of upper lobe pulmonary vessels. Mitral stenosis is one of the cardiac causes for elevated pulmonary venous pressure, although it has become relatively uncommon. The well-known radiographic signs of pulmonary edema are cardiomegaly, pleural effusions, and vascular congestion. Interstitial edema can be seen with blurring of the margins of blood vessels around the bronchial wall—called *peribronchial cuffing*—and in the subpleural position—called *Kerley B lines*. As capillary pressure rises, accumulated fluid in the interstitium adds to the interstitial pressure, forcing fluid into the alveolar space. Differentiation between pulmonary edema due to increased circular blood volume and that due to a failing left ventricle can be made on the basis of measurement of the vascular pedicle if the technique is not flawed. The radiographic differentiation of hydrostatic pulmonary edema from increased capillary permeability is also difficult. The criteria used are cardiac size, vascular distribution, and measurement of the vascular pedicle; this test has a predictive value of 75%. Some authors believe that the best sign of hydrostatic pulmonary edema is an abnormal right costophrenic angle containing Kerley B lines, subpleural edema, and pleural effusion. Those patients who have increased capillary permeability frequently have normal right costophrenic angles. The other most useful sign is the presence of an air bronchogram in increased capillary permeability edema and its absence in hydrostatic edema.

The diagnosis of mitral stenosis is associated with a diastolic rumble on physical exam. The first heart sound is loud and there is no clubbing or koilonychia. Mitral stenosis may be complicated by atrial arrhythmias, hemoptysis secondary to left ventricular failure, or endocarditis. Atrial myxoma is not a complication but may mimic signs and symptoms of mitral stenosis. The radiographic sign suggestive of an atrial enlargement is a widened carinal angle.

123–124. The answers are 123-b, 124-d. The clinical syndrome described best fits the diagnosis of atrial septal defect with secondary pulmonary hypertension. The chest radiograph is consistent with pulmonary hypertension. Other options are inappropriate. The next diagnostic step would be to do an echocardiogram.

CHEST WALL AND SKELETAL DEFORMITIES

DIRECTIONS: Each item below contains a question or incomplete statement followed by suggested responses. Select the **one best** response to each question.

Items 125–127

A 34-year-old truck driver with a recent history of MVA complains of dull, aching left-sided chest pain and shortness of breath. Physical examination: pulse 100 bpm; temperature 99°F; respirations 24/min; blood pressure 120/80 mm Hg. The patient is in mild distress with left chest wall tenderness. Lung exam reveals faint crackles in the left lung field but is otherwise normal. ABGs on RA: pH 7.5; P_{CO_2} 32 mm Hg; P_{O_2} 87 mm Hg. Chest radiograph is shown below in Fig. 70.

125. What is the most likely diagnosis?

a. Pulmonary embolism
b. Pneumothorax
c. Left-sided rib fractures
d. Pleurisy

126. What is the next management option?

a. Antibiotics
b. Pain relief with chest stabilization
c. Chest tube placement
d. Anticoagulants

127. Complications of this condition may include

a. Pneumonia/atelectasis
b. Cerebral abscess
c. Chronic dyspnea and restrictive lung disease
d. Fat embolism

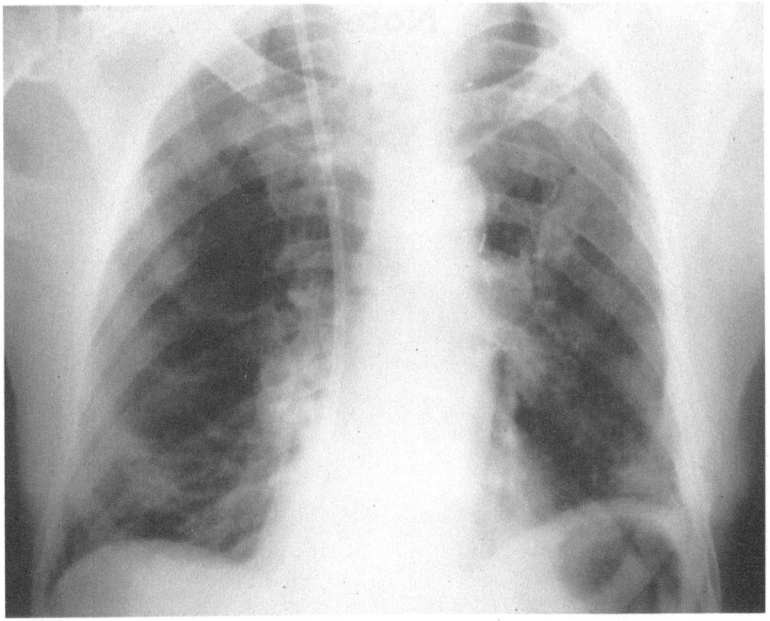

Fig. 70

Notes

Items 128–130

A 78-year-old female nonsmoker with a history of osteoporosis is seen with the chief complaint of increased exertional dyspnea. Physical examination: pulse 110 bpm; temperature normal; respirations 24/min; blood pressure 110/60 mm Hg. The patient is frail-looking, with decreased respiratory excursion on chest exam. Heart exam reveals normal sinus rhythm with grade 2/6 systolic murmur and loud P_2 sound. Laboratory data: Hb 14.2 g/dL; Hct 42%; WBCs 9.0/μL. ABGs on room air: pH 7.38; P_{CO_2} 45 mm Hg; P_{O_2} 56 mm Hg. Chest radiographs are shown below in Fig. 71.

128. What is the most likely diagnosis?
a. Kyphoscoliosis
b. Interstitial lung disease
c. Aortic dissection
d. Hiatal hernia

129. PFT of this patient will show
a. Reversible obstructive defect
b. Restriction with normal DLCO
c. Restriction with decreased DLCO
d. Normal

130. The ABG abnormality seen is due to
a. V/Q mismatch
b. Alveolar hypoventilation
c. Diffusion defect
d. Patent foramen ovale

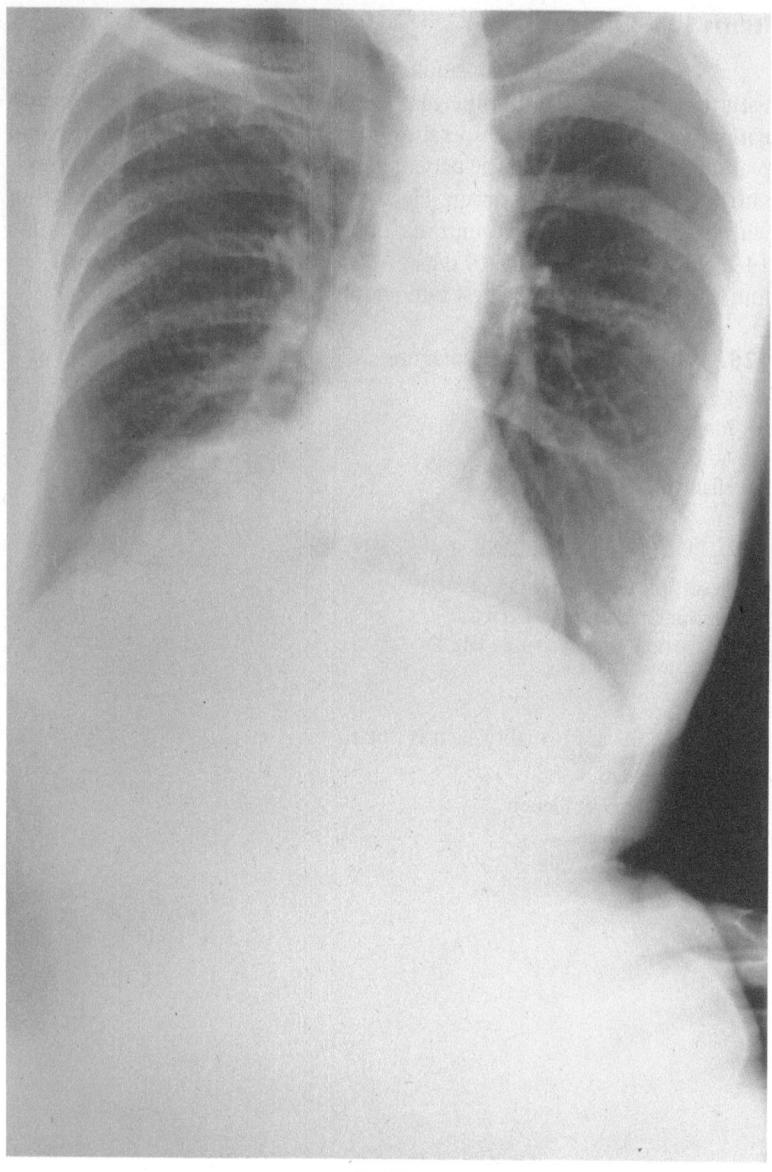

Fig. 71a

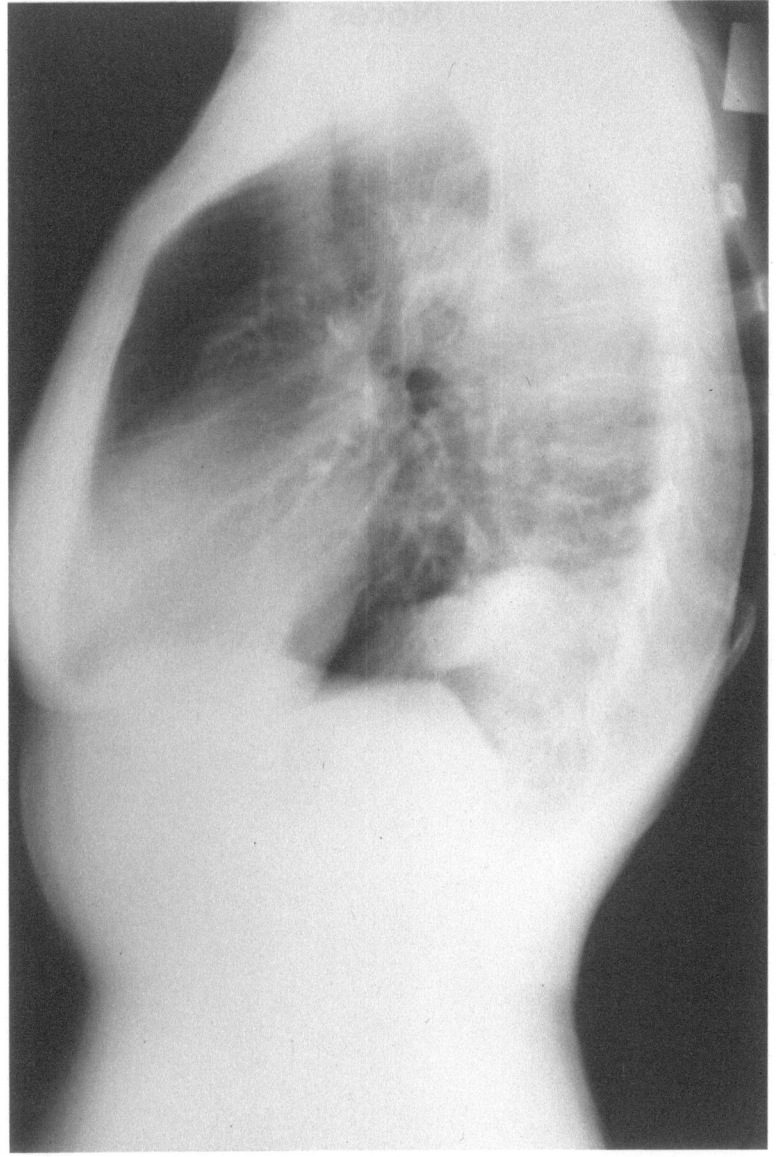

Fig. 71b

Notes

Chest Wall and Skeletal Deformities

Items 131–133

A 38-year-old man is seen with a 2-day history of fever, postnasal drip, cough, and nonspecific chest discomfort. He has been treated for TB in the past for 18 mo. On physical examination, his lungs are clear to auscultation and heart exam reveals a midsystolic click. Sputum tests are negative for acid-fast bacilli. Chest x-rays are shown below in Fig. 72.

131. What is the most likely cause of this patient's symptoms?
a. Mitral valve prolapse
b. Reactivation of TB
c. Costochondritis
d. Acute upper respiratory tract illness

132. This x-ray picture is characteristically associated with the following pulmonary function test abnormality:
a. Severe restrictive defect
b. Mild obstruction
c. Normal
d. Mixed obstructive and restrictive dysfunction

133. The patient is concerned about his x-ray. The next management step is
a. Consult thoracic surgeon for corrective surgery
b. Treat with bronchodilator
c. Perform incentive spirometry
d. Treat the acute symptoms and reassure the patient

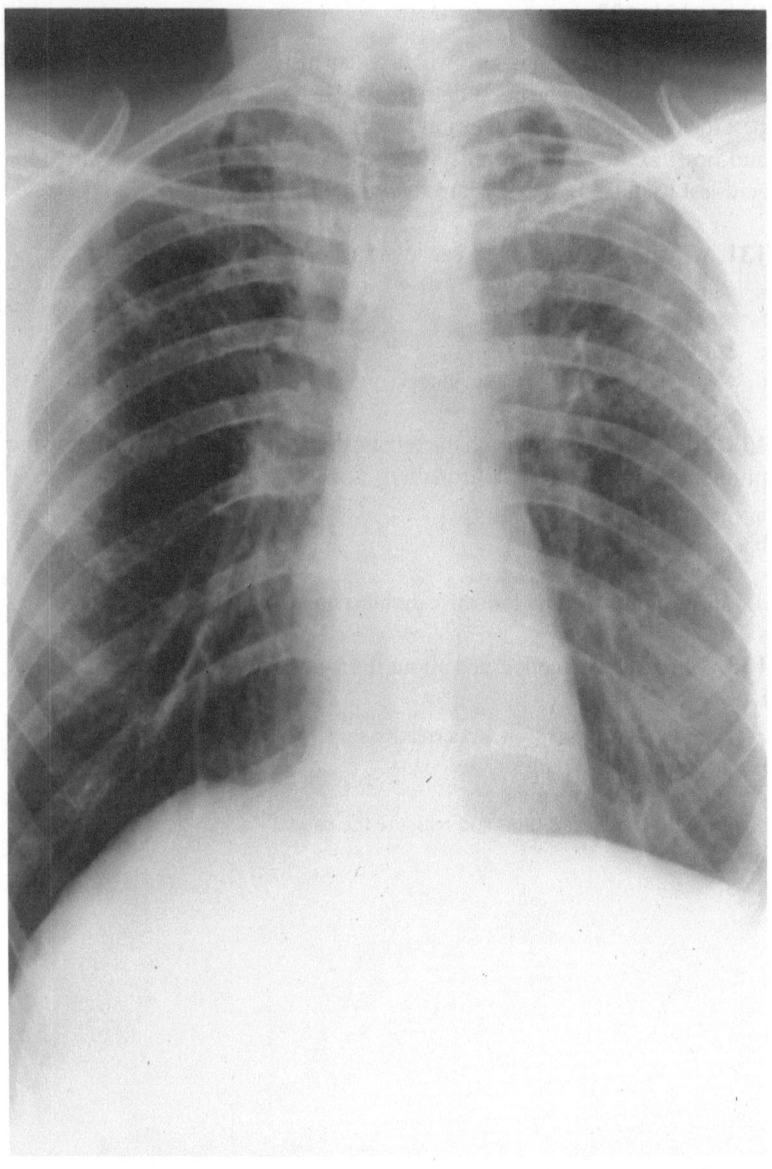

Fig. 72a

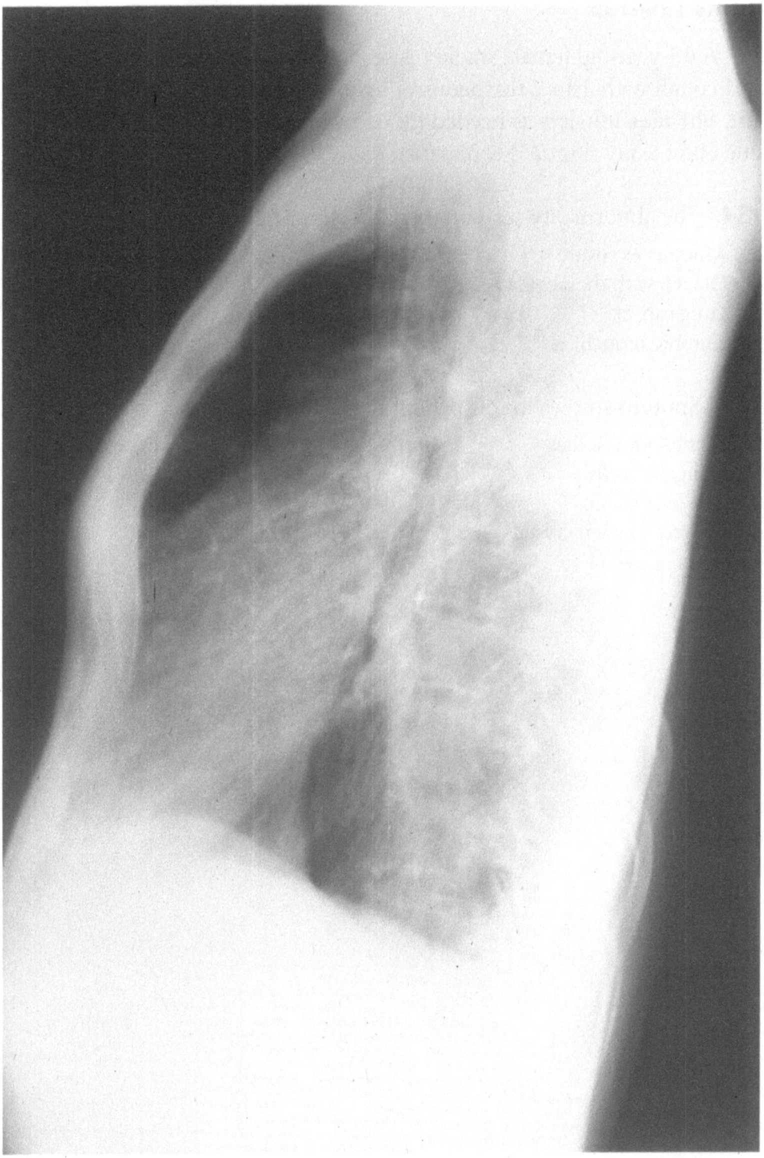

Fig. 72b

Items 134–135

A 68-year-old female smoker is seen in the ER due to mild hemoptysis and cough with 1 to 2 teaspoons of light-green sputum production in the A.M. She uses inhalers as needed for occasional shortness of breath. A routine chest x-ray (Fig. 73) is obtained.

134. The abnormality seen on the CXR is most likely due to

a. Asbestos exposure
b. Old TB with thoracoplasty
c. Lung cancer
d. Chronic bronchitis

135. Sputum studies in this patient may show

a. Ferruginous bodies
b. Malignant cells
c. Acid-fast bacilli
d. Charcot-Leyden crystals

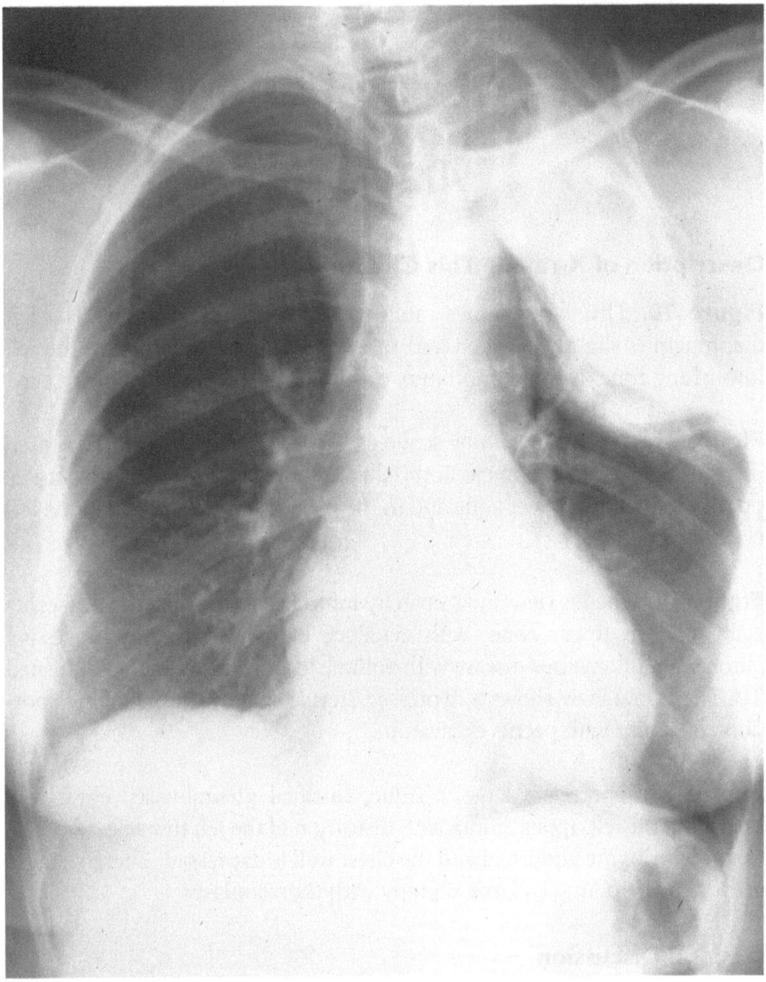

Fig. 73

CHEST WALL AND SKELETAL DEFORMITIES

Answers

Description of X-rays in This Chapter

Figure 70. This x-ray shows multiple left-sided rib fractures. The left diaphragm is slightly elevated and there is a minimal infiltrate in the left lower lung zone. No pneumothorax or significant pleural effusion is seen.

Figure 71. These views show scoliosis of the thoracic spine with marked displacement of the thoracic aorta shadow giving a distorted soft tissue opacity in the right lower zone and in the posterior mediastinum in the lateral projection.

Figure 72. The PA view shows patchy infiltrates in the upper zones, especially the left upper zone, with evidence of hilar retraction suggesting chronic granulomatous disease with volume loss. This is seen in old, treated TB. The lateral view shows a depressed sternal shadow in the inferior portion consistent with pectus excavatum.

Figure 73. There is a large, opaque, calcified pleural-based chest wall opacity in the left upper thorax with distortion of the left thoracic cage. The upper left ribs are abnormal and the chest wall is depressed. These changes are a sequela to lung collapse therapy with thoracoplasty.

General Discussion

The chest wall includes the thoracic cage and the neuromuscular tissues within it. Disease and deformities may arise from all components. Physical examination often detects these abnormalities, but imaging techniques are often needed to evaluate their extent. Chest wall lesions appear on a chest x-ray with an "extra pleural sign." These lesions have a convex inward smooth border, and their greatest diameter is in the midportion of the lesion. They tend to make an acute angle with the chest wall, and underlying ribs are involved. Infections as well as tumors may involve the chest wall and the surrounding tissue. Chest wall lesions account for 2% of all primary tumors; primary soft tissue tumors are more common than primary bony tumors. Bronchogenic tumors may involve the chest wall by direct extension with infiltration of the surrounding tissue.

Specific Discussion

125–127. The answers are 125-c, 126-b, 127-a. When rib fractures are present, patients usually experience pain. When several ribs are fractured, the respiratory status may become compromised. *Flail chest* describes a condition with paradoxical movement, especially of the lower chest wall. During inspiration, when the thorax normally expands in all directions, the negative intrapleural pressures will cause the unstable portion of the chest wall to draw in. Similarly, on expiration, the unstable portion of the chest wall moves outward. This results in diminished effectiveness of breathing, and the pain from rib fracture may lead to splinting of the chest wall, thus impairing ventilation. Complications such as atelectasis and pulmonary infections can occur. If large areas of the chest wall are unstable, mechanical ventilation may be considered, as this provides a form of internal fixation of the chest wall. Chronic residual effects of flail chest are uncommon. Rib fractures are a common result of chest trauma, and a chest radiograph is needed as a follow-up for complications of these fractures such as pneumothorax, atelectasis, or pneumonia. Intercostal nerve blocks provide substantial relief of pain.

128–130. The answers are 128-a, 129-b, 130-a. Kyphoscoliosis is a combination of excessive anterior and posterior lateral curvature of the thoracic spine. The abnormal curvature may be laterally dominant as a scoliosis or posteriorly as kyphosis. Deformity of a sufficient degree leads to symptoms and signs referable to the lungs and heart. This occurs in less than 3% of those with abnormal curvature. About 80% of cases of scoliosis are idiopathic, with no clear cause identified. The disease is classified into three types—infantile, juvenile, and adult-onset—depending on age at presentation. Congenital forms of kyphoscoliosis are related to other abnormalities of the thoracic spine such as hemivertebra or deformities of the spine associated with neurofibromatosis, muscular dystrophy, Friedreich's ataxia, acquired neuromuscular disease associated with poliomyelitis, or infection of the spine with tuberculosis. Major complications of severe kyphoscoliosis are pulmonary artery hypertension, cor pulmonale, and chronic respiratory failure. Pulmonary hypertension is due to chronic hypoxemia, which is secondary to V/Q mismatch. Restrictive lung defect is seen on pulmonary function tests, and diffusion abnormality is uncommon. Manipulations of the spine result more in cosmetic improvement than change in pulmonary function. Nasal BiPAP may help reduce arterial P_{CO_2} with increasing P_{O_2} and therefore improve pulmonary artery pressures. Consideration of nocturnal ventilation should be given to all patients with kyphoscoliosis and recurrent respiratory failure.

131–133. The answers are 131-d, 132-c, 133-d. The symptoms in this patient are due to an acute upper respiratory tract infection. The midsystolic click is most likely an incidental finding and does not represent mitral valve prolapse syndrome. Typical TB infection is unlikely in this patient previously treated for *Mycobacterium avium* disease and with a negative sputum smear now. The skeletal deformity shown is pectus excavatum, which does not cause costochondritis. Pectus excavatum is characterized by an inward depression of the sternum and lower costal cartilage with normal manubrium and first and second ribs. In extreme cases this may cause displacement of the heart and mediastinal structures; the heart shadow may appear enlarged and the right hilum indistinct on the PA view. The lateral radiograph confirms the depressed sternum. Respiratory symptoms are uncommon, and pulmonary functions are normal. Surgical correction is seldom indicated. Pectus carinatum is characterized by an outward protrusion of the sternum due to the costal cartilages and is usually congenital. However, it can be associated with chronic severe asthma.

134–135. The answers are 134-b, 135-c. Thoracoplasty is the excision of substantial segments of the bony thorax to reduce its size. The indication for thoracoplasty in this case was unilateral cavitary pulmonary tuberculosis that had not responded to other forms of treatment. Occasionally, thoracoplasty is still done to obliterate empyema cavities. Following thoracoplasty, large tuberculous cavities heal by organization of granulation tissue and the contracted tissue becomes encased in a thick pleural membrane. Associated pleural calcification and thickening are seen.

DIAPHRAGMATIC LESIONS

DIRECTIONS: Each item below contains a question or incomplete statement followed by suggested responses. Select the **one best** response to each question.

136. A 64-year-old woman with a longstanding diagnosis of mixed connective tissue disorder and pulmonary fibrosis is admitted with symptoms of recent increase in postprandial retrosternal distress, heartburn, and nocturnal cough. Her ECG shows nonspecific T-wave changes and she finds minimal relief of her symptoms with sublingual NTG. On examination, she is not in any acute distress and is afebrile. Chest exam reveals bilateral crackles. CXR is shown in Fig. 74. The cause of this patient's acute symptoms may be

a. Large hiatal hernia
b. Mediastinal abscess
c. Pneumopericardium
d. Ileus

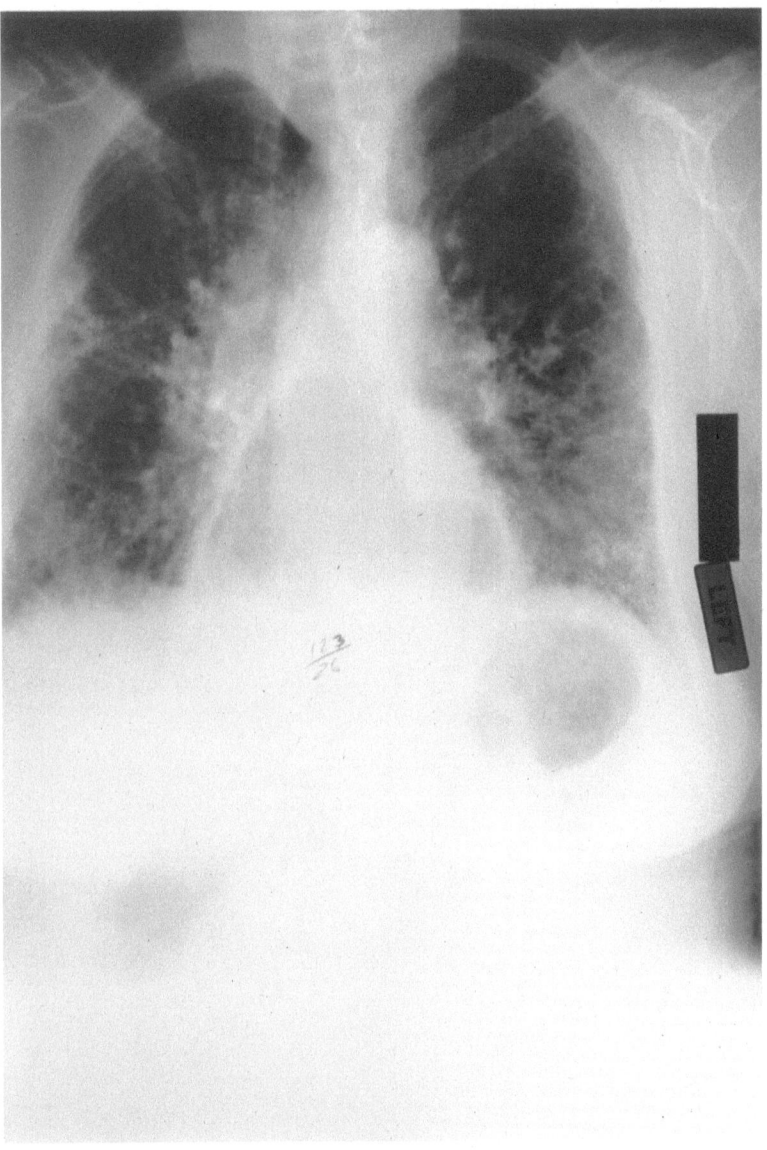

Fig. 74

Notes

Items 137-138

A 40-year-old woman is referred for evaluation of a "mass" seen on a chest x-ray. Chest x-rays (Fig. 75) are shown below.

137. The diagnosis is
a. Bronchogenic cyst
b. Hernia through the foramen of Bochdalek
c. Hydatid cyst
d. Loculated pleural effusion

138. This finding
a. Is more common on the left
b. Is usually associated with severe symptoms
c. Requires immediate surgery
d. Cannot be confirmed by a barium swallow

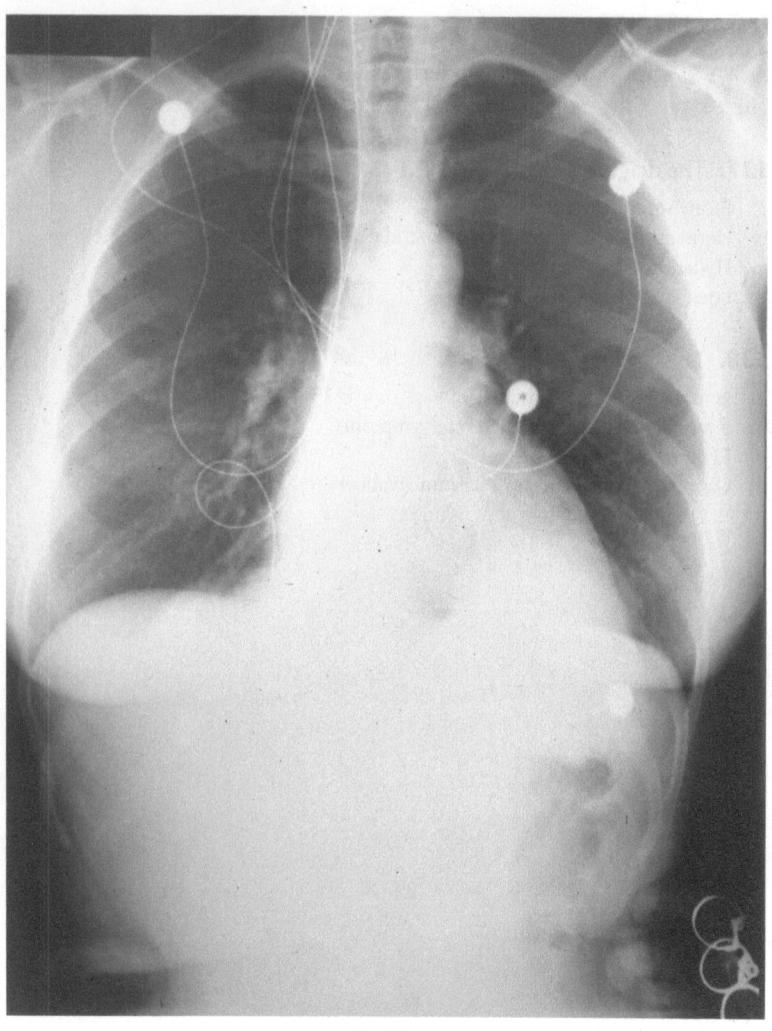

Fig. 75a

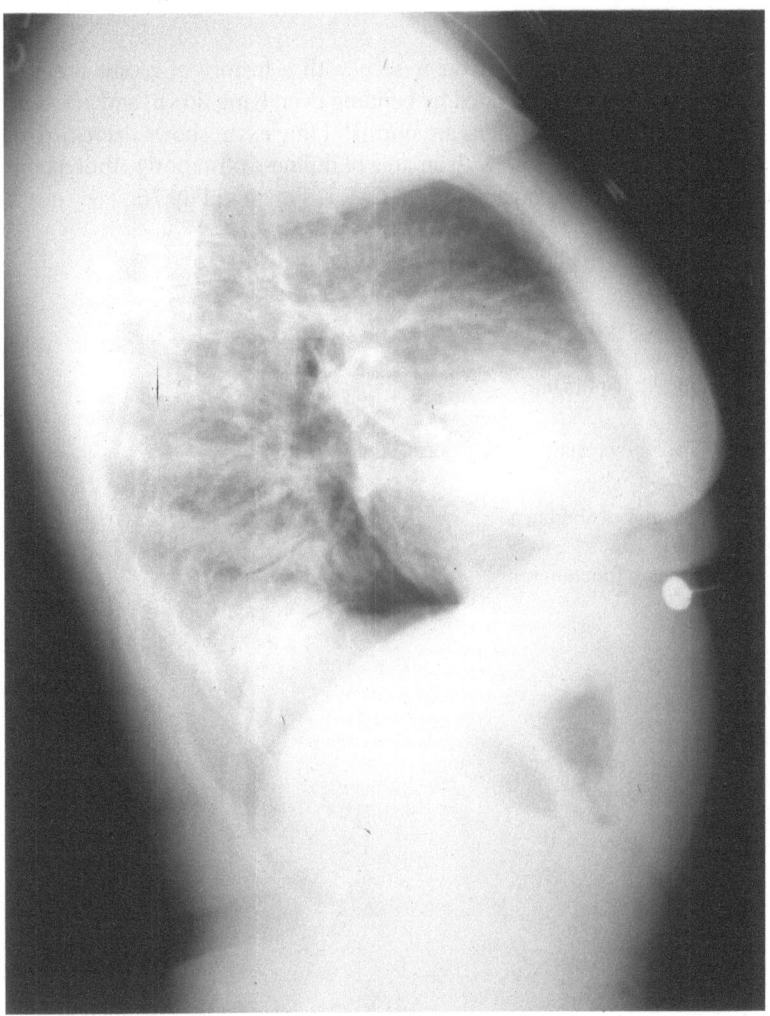

Fig. 75b

Items 139–140

A 37-year-old truck driver is seen with a history of recent onset of shortness of breath aggravated by bending over, lying down, and exertion. On physical exam, vital signs are normal. Lung exam shows decreased air movement at the left base with an area of dullness posteriorly. Abdomen is soft without palpable organomegaly. CXR is shown in Fig. 76.

139. The abnormality on the CXR is most likely due to
a. LLL atelectasis
b. Enlarged spleen
c. Subphrenic abscess
d. Paralyzed diaphragm

140. The above diagnosis can best be confirmed by
a. Sniff test
b. Ultrasound of abdomen
c. Bronchoscopy
d. Pulmonary function test

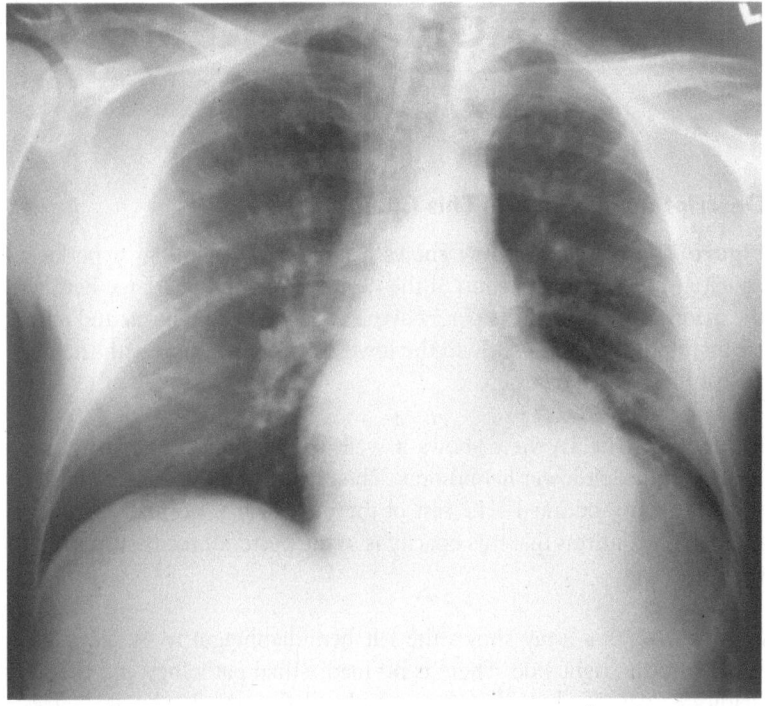

Fig. 76

Diaphragmatic Lesions

Answers

Description of X-rays in This Chapter

Figure 74. This chest x-ray shows a large, air-containing, hyperlucent opacity in the middle portion of the thorax representing a large hernia in the mediastinum. The lung parenchyma shows increased linear and reticular markings, predominantly in the lower zones, consistent with the diagnosis of interstitial disease.

Figure 75. The PA view shows a well-defined and clearly marginated opacity in the left lower hemithorax. The cardiac and diaphragmatic shadows are clearly outlined. The rest of the lung field is normal. The lateral radiograph confirms that this opacity is in the posterior mediastinum abutting the spine.

Figure 76. This x-ray shows the left hemidiaphragm to be elevated in relation to the right side. There is no mediastinal pathology and the lung fields are clear. The hyperlucent gas shadow below the diaphragm suggests that there is no subdiaphragmatic pathology.

General Discussion

The diaphragm is the most important muscle of respiration. Abnormalities are infrequent. Functional impairment of the diaphragm is reflected on the chest radiograph by changes in its relative position. Defects noted in the diaphragm are bilateral elevation, unilateral elevation, eventration, and displacement due to an intraabdominal process. A subpulmonic effusion may appear as an elevation or alteration in the diaphragm contour. Tumors are rare. Trauma may result in various degrees of tearing with herniation of abdominal viscera. Congenital or acquired defects occur most commonly at the insertions into the chest wall. Evaluation of these disorders would require fluoroscopy to assess diaphragm function, paralysis, or weakness. Respiratory insufficiency may occur due to diaphragmatic involvement.

Specific Discussion

136. The answer is a. The symptoms described are due to an acid reflux disorder, and the chest x-ray shows a large hiatal hernia. Hiatal hernia represents herniation of the stomach through the esophageal hiatus and is frequently found in adults. It occurs as an oval retrocardiac mass, most often with an air-fluid level, and is due to laxity, stretching, and widening of the hiatus. Obesity and increased intraabdominal pressures are contributing factors. The majority of hernias spontaneously reduce and are called *sliding hernias*. A paraesophageal hernia occurs when the stomach herniates next to the distal esophagus. Patients may be asymptomatic or may have symptoms of reflux.

137–138. The answers are 137-b, 138-a. Diaphragmatic hernias are common. Congenital diaphragmatic hernia occurs as a result of the failure of the closure of the pleural peritoneal fold during the first trimester. It is more common on the left side and is associated with other congenital anomalies. Communication between the abdomen and the thorax may allow abdominal contents to enter the chest.

Bochdalek hernias are the most common congenital diaphragmatic hernias. They occur in 1 in 2200 to 2500 live births, and the ratio of left- to right-sided diaphragmatic defects is approximately 9:1. These hernias are located in the posterolateral portion of the diaphragm. This is thought to be due to the fact that the liver affords protection on the right side. They appear as soft tissue masses arising from the posterior aspect of the hemidiaphragm on the radiograph. Small defects contain fat; larger defects can contain stomach, spleen, kidney, or liver. If small, Bochdalek hernias may remain undetected until later on in life since they are almost always asymptomatic. Computerized tomography is able to demonstrate not only large, clinically symptomatic diaphragmatic hernias in newborns, but also small, clinically silent defects in adults. On a lateral chest film, a single, smooth focal bulge is seen centered approximately 4 to 5 cm anterior to the posterior diaphragmatic insertion.

Morgagni hernias are anteriomedial and more common on the right side. Herniation occurs through the sternal costal area due to failed union of the sternum and the fibrous tendons of the diaphragm. These hernias are associated with obesity and usually contain fat. The transverse colon is more involved than the stomach or the bowel. Although most patients are asymptomatic, some may complain of respiratory or epigastric pressure or pain.

139–140. The answers are 139-d, 140-a. Unilateral elevation of the hemidiaphragm can be seen as a result of an enlargement or displacement of an abdominal organ, a subpulmonic process such as effusion, loss of volume of the lung with lobar atelectasis or surgical resection, or hemidiaphragmatic paralysis. Diaphragmatic paralysis results from interruption of the phrenic nerve supply to the diaphragm. The most common cause is malignancy, such as bronchogenic carcinoma, or postsurgical trauma. Twenty percent of patients who undergo open heart surgery sustain injury to the phrenic nerve. Other causes of diaphragmatic paralysis include polio, herpes, infections, lead poisoning, pulmonary infarctions, pneumonia, mediastinitis, and pericarditis. The diagnosis of unilateral paralysis of the diaphragm is suggested by the finding of an elevated hemidiaphragm on the chest x-ray. With diaphragmatic paralysis, the negative pleural pressure tends to pull the paralyzed diaphragm upward. Normally the right diaphragm is about 3 cm higher than the left. Confirmation of diaphragmatic paralysis is established by the sniff test. In this test the diaphragm is observed fluoroscopically as the patient sniffs. The normal diaphragm is moved downward during the sniff maneuver as the diaphragmatic muscles contract. A paralyzed diaphragm moves paradoxically upward because of negative pleural pressure. Patients with paralyzed diaphragms may be asymptomatic or may complain of dyspnea on lying down or with exertion. With complete paralysis, vital capacity and total lung capacity may be reduced about 25% from the baseline, and the maximum inspiratory pressure is reduced to about 40%.

Lines/Devices/Complications in ICU

Chest Radiology

DIRECTIONS: Each item below contains a question or incomplete statement followed by suggested responses. Select the **one best** response to each question.

Items 141–142

A 64-year-old woman is admitted to the ICU with the clinical diagnosis of acute respiratory distress syndrome (ARDS) secondary to pneumonia. She requires intubation and mechanical ventilation. On the second ICU day, she is difficult to ventilate, requiring increased airway pressures. On physical examination, vital signs are: pulse 159 bpm; temperature 100°F; blood pressure 90/56 mm Hg. Lung exam reveals diffuse crackles, and the patient has a palpable crunch on exam of her chest wall and abdomen. Chest radiograph is shown below in Fig. 77.

141. What is the most likely diagnosis?

a. Nosocomial infection
b. Pneumomediastinum
c. Pneumopericardium
d. Gas gangrene

142. What will you do next?

a. Place a chest tube
b. Change antibiotics
c. Perform an open thoracotomy
d. Continue management, minimizing volutrauma

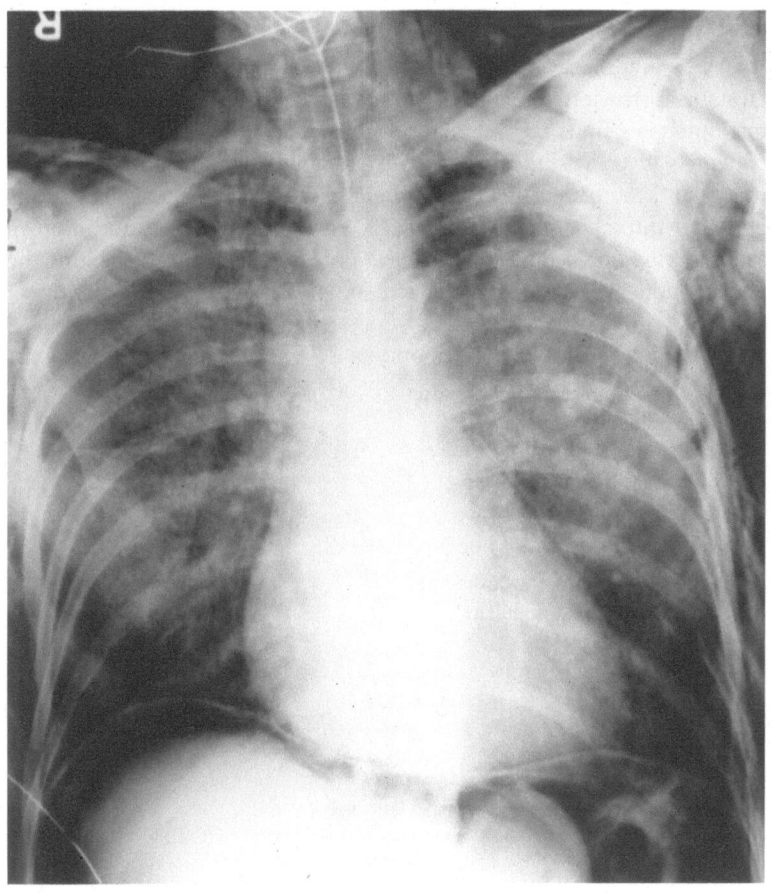

Fig. 77

Items 143–144

A 40-year-old woman admitted with fever, chills, and changing mental status is transferred to the ICU with a clinical suspicion of sepsis. Examination shows sinus tachycardia, no murmur, and clear lung fields. The patient is given IV fluids aggressively for hydration. Blood cultures are drawn and the patient is placed on antibiotics. Subcutaneous heparin is given for thromboembolic prophylaxis. As the patient does not improve satisfactorily, a procedure is performed. One hour after this procedure, the patient suddenly develops moderate hemoptysis. A CXR (Fig. 78) is done.

143. The likely cause of the hemoptysis is
a. Silent unrecognized mitral stenosis
b. Acute pulmonary edema
c. Complication of heparin therapy
d. Pulmonary infarction

144. The next step should be
a. Perform an urgent echocardiogram
b. Administer protamine sulfate
c. Start inotropic agents
d. Withdraw the catheter

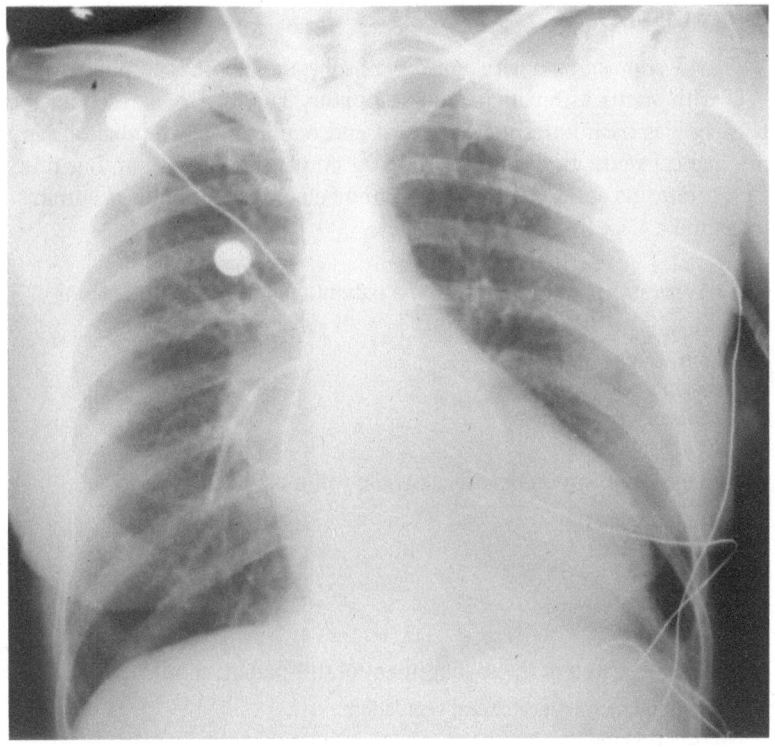

Fig. 78

Items 145–147

A 43-year-old man with a history of substance abuse is admitted to the ICU with status asthmaticus and respiratory failure. Upon reaching the ICU, he has a cardiorespiratory arrest and requires CPR, intubation, and mechanical ventilation. BP was 160/100 mm Hg on admission, but post-CPR it remains at 80/60 mm Hg. An immediate IV fluid bolus is administered and a CXR (Fig. 79) is done.

145. What is a possible cause of the patient's persistent hypotension?
a. Pneumonia
b. Severe status asthmaticus
c. Tension pneumothorax
d. Pulmonary embolism

146. Physical exam on the affected side will most likely reveal
a. Pleural friction rub
b. Severe wheezing
c. Area of egophony
d. Absent breath sounds

147. The next step in the management of this patient should be
a. Discontinuation of mechanical ventilation
b. Anticoagulant therapy
c. Chest tube placement
d. Inotropic agents

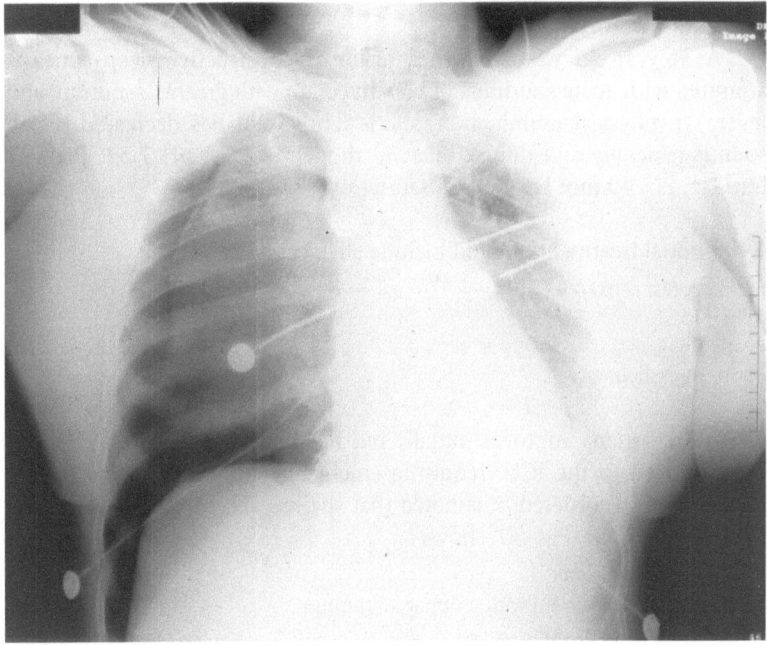

Fig. 79

Items 148–150

A 36-year-old woman with a history of obstructive sleep apnea is admitted with acute shortness of breath, cough with greenish sputum, and fever. On physical examination, she is febrile and has decreased breath sounds generally and diffuse bilateral rhonchi. ABGs: pH 7.32; P_{CO_2} 47 mm Hg; P_{O_2} 65 mm Hg with O_2 saturation 87%.

148. Initial treatments should include all except
a. β agonist aerosol Rx
b. O_2 Rx
c. Antibiotics
d. IV theophylline

149. The patient improves initially but has a respiratory arrest as she is being moved to the ICU, requiring emergency endotracheal intubation. While a CXR is ordered, it is noted that she has absent breath sounds on the left side. CXR (Fig. 80) shows
a. Left pneumothorax
b. Pneumomediastinum with esophageal rupture
c. Left pleural effusion
d. Atelectasis

150. The next step to be taken should be
a. Surgical consult
b. Pleural tap
c. Repositioning of the endotracheal tube
d. Chest tube placement

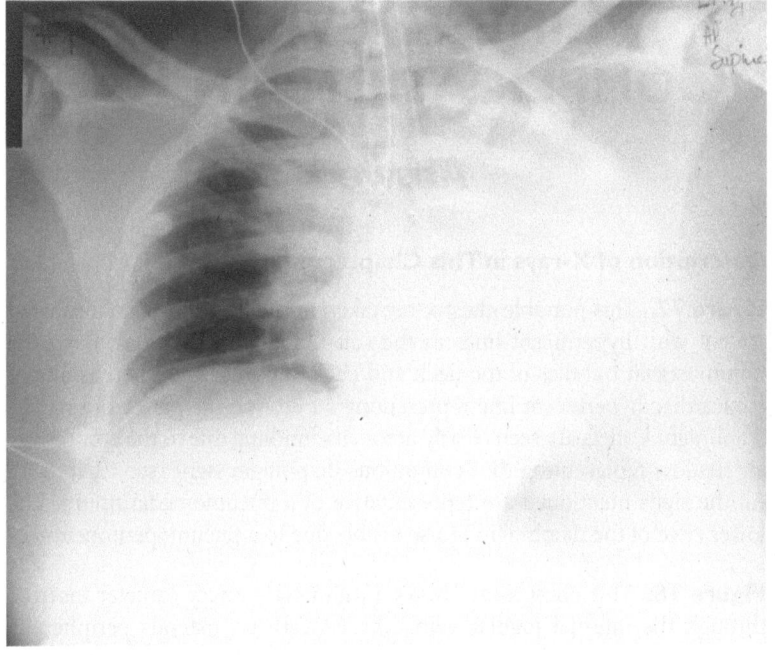

Fig. 80

LINES/DEVICES/ COMPLICATIONS IN ICU

Answers

Description of X-rays in This Chapter

Figure 77. This portable chest x-ray taken in the ICU shows an intubated patient with hyperlucent lines in the soft tissue with striations along the fibromuscular bundles of the neck and chest musculature. There is a faint paracardiac hyperlucent line representing air around the pericardium. The diaphragm leaflets are seen clearly across the midline due to the contrasting air shadow representing the "continuous diaphragm sign" (see Chap. 15). All the signs mentioned are representative of a pneumomediastinum. The lower edge of the diaphragm is also visible due to a pneumoperitoneum.

Figure 78. This chest x-ray shows a pulmonary artery catheter inserted through the internal jugular vein. The PA catheter extends peripherally beyond the right ventricular shadow and past the main pulmonary artery branches into the subsegmental vessels.

Figure 79. The patient is intubated and being monitored. The mediastinum is shifted to the left with loss of volume of the left lung. The left diaphragm is elevated. The right lung field is hyperlucent and there is an area of further relative increased hyperlucency with a distinct medial border. This is called the visceral pleural line. The right costophrenic angle is acute and very deep; this is called the "deep sulcus sign." The presence of contralateral mediastinal shift, lowered diaphragm, and widened interspaces on the right suggests a tension pneumothorax.

Figure 80. The chest radiograph shows a homogeneous opacity occupying the left hemithorax with no air bronchograms. The left heart border and left diaphragm are not seen, consistent with left lung atelectasis. The right upper zone parahilar area is also partially opacified, suggesting partial right upper lobe atelectasis. An endotracheal tube is seen extending down to the right intermediate bronchus.

General Discussion

Management of the critically ill patient has become complex due to the use of monitoring and life support devices. The physician needs to be aware of the common life support devices used, such as endotracheal tubes, tracheostomy tubes, flow-directed balloon catheters, central venous lines, and chest tubes. Opacities seen after cardiac bypass and valve replacement surgery need to be recognized. Some of the complications arising from the placement of these devices may lead to pulmonary complications such as pneumothorax, alveolar hemorrhage, and atelectasis. Changes on the chest radiograph may therefore represent a combination of opacities related to the primary process and interventional techniques.

Specific Discussion

141–142. The answers are 141-b, 142-d. Alveolar rupture with increased alveolar-interstitial space gradient can cause pneumomediastinum and subcutaneous emphysema. Subcutaneous emphysema may occur after trauma such as esophageal rupture with direct introduction of air in the mediastinum. It can also occur where there is abdominal and thoracic muscular contraction against a closed glottis. Infection with a gas-forming organism can cause subcutaneous gas formation. Inflammatory bronchiolitis or overinflated alveoli due to mechanical ventilation can cause alveolar rupture, especially if there is airway obstruction with air moving along the bronchovascular sheaths. Pneumomediastinum refers to abnormal air collection within the mediastinum. Air can dissect into the mediastinum from areas of the neck and thorax or from the GI tract or lungs. Pathologically there is continuity between the periarterial and the peribronchial interstitium when an alveolar rupture occurs, creating an air collection within the interstitial connective tissues. Patient-related factors that are found to predispose to volutrauma include lung disease that weakens alveolar walls, such as COPD and necrotizing pneumonia. Mediastinal air accumulates and then decompresses into the subcutaneous tissues and the retroperitoneal areas. Later, mediastinal pleura may rupture, resulting in a pneumothorax. The Hamman sign, a crunching sound synchronous with the cardiac cycle, is seen in 40% to 50% of patients with pneumomediastinum. When the pneumomediastinum extends caudally, it shows a so-called "continuous diaphragm sign." Treatment is usually conservative, with attempts to reduce airway resistance with bronchodilator therapy and minimize tidal volume and plateau pressure.

143–144. The answers are 143-d, 144-d. The patient presents with sepsis and septic shock. It is important to determine the fluid status of the patient, especially if no improvement is noted with initial fluid challenge. The procedure performed was a placement of a pulmonary artery catheter to determine the capillary wedge pressure. The PA catheter in this case extended peripherally into the small vessels and thereby caused pulmonary infarction. The hemoptysis represents that complication, and withdrawal of the catheter is of utmost priority. Other options outlined are inappropriate or inapplicable.

145–147. The answers are 145-c, 146-d, 147-c. A pneumothorax is air within the pleural space and is a common sequela to chest trauma. In the ICU, with the patient in a supine position, the usual apical distribution of air in the pleural space and the visceral pleural line indicating the edge of the collapsed lung may not be as evident. Air accumulates medially around the midchest region when the thoracic cage is most anterior. In this case, the hyperlucent area in the lateral chest and the costophrenic angle clearly indicates air in the pleural space. The "deep sulcus sign" is a pneumothorax seen in a supine position at the costophrenic or cardiophrenic angle, both of which may represent elevated points of the thoracic cage. The clinical history shows that the patient suddenly decompensated. The low BP is due to decreased venous return. In a pneumothorax, the breath sounds are absent on the affected side and a chest tube is needed to evacuate the pleural air, reduce the positive intrapleural pressure, and expand the lung.

148–150. The answers are 148-d, 149-d, 150-c. This patient was admitted with symptoms of pneumonia with hypoxemia and respiratory acidosis. Initial treatment should include controlled oxygen therapy, antibiotics, and aerosolized bronchodilator therapy. IV theophylline is not considered standard practice and is not a first-line drug for bronchospasm. During CPR and resuscitation, traumatic pneumothorax and pneumomediastinum can occur. The CXR shows left-sided atelectasis with the endotracheal tube placed distally in the right intermediate bronchus. Correct positioning of the tube above the carina should be the first step in this case.

Pediatric Cases

Chest Radiology

DIRECTIONS: Each item below contains a question or incomplete statement followed by suggested responses. Select the **one best** response to each question.

Items 151–152

An 8-year-old girl is brought to the clinic by her mother. The child has high-grade fever, cough, and increased irritability. Further history reveals that the child's grandmother, who lives with the family, was diagnosed with pulmonary tuberculosis. A chest x-ray (Fig. 81) is done.

151. Regarding the diagnosis based on the clinical history and chest x-ray shown, choose the most correct answer.
a. Most infected children have severe symptoms.
b. Initial chest x-ray is usually diagnostic.
c. Late clinical manifestation may include chronic otorrhea.
d. A multiple puncture test should be used for diagnosis in children.

152. Other x-ray presentation may include
a. Pleural effusion
b. Pectus excavatum
c. Mycetoma
d. Pneumomediastinum

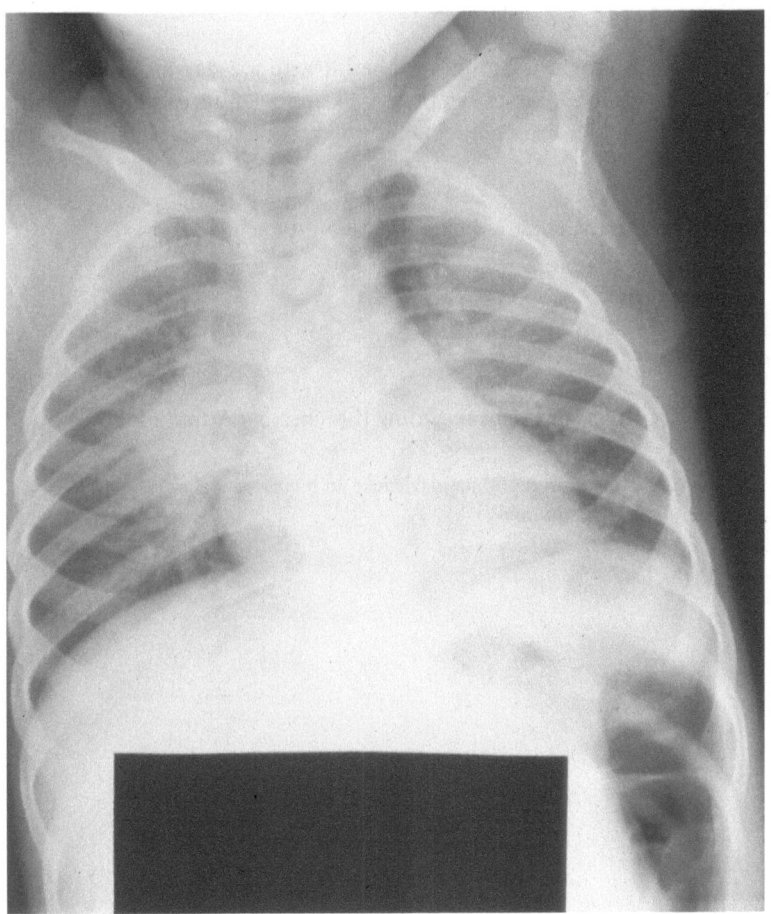

Fig. 81

Items 153–154

A 4-year-old girl is brought to the ER with a 2-day history of cough and upper respiratory tract symptoms. Examination reveals bilateral otitis media. The mother insists on obtaining a chest radiograph, which is done (see Fig. 82).

153. Based on the chest radiograph, the most likely diagnosis is
a. Respiratory syncytial virus
b. Normal variant
c. Lymphoma
d. Primary tuberculosis

154. The correct statement regarding this chest x-ray finding is
a. It increases with age.
b. Chemotherapy for lymphoma may cause an increase in its size.
c. Carcinoma is common.
d. It is usually symmetrical.

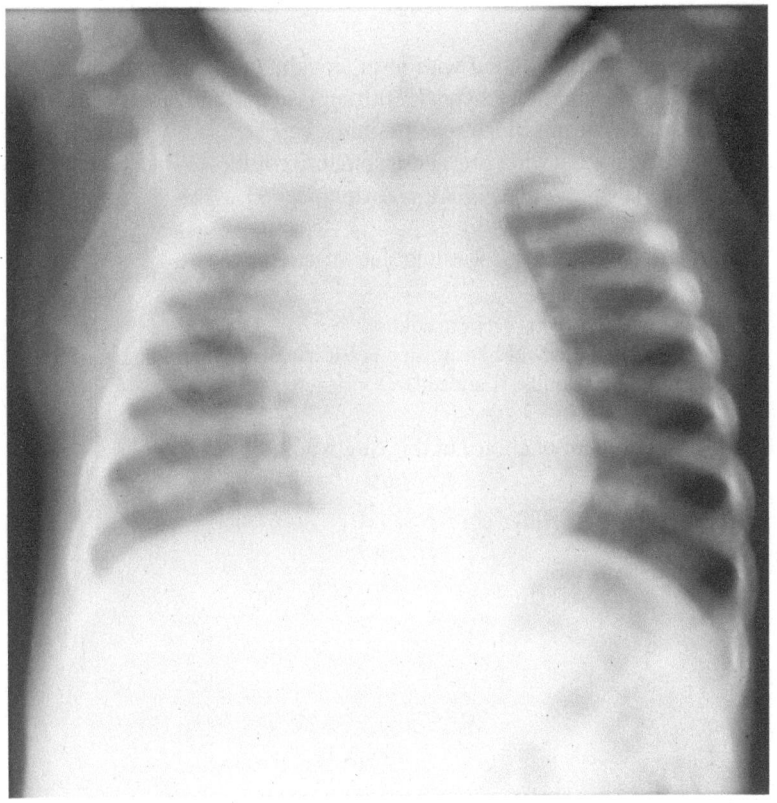

Fig. 82

Items 155-156

A 2-year-old is admitted with fever, cough, and bilateral earache. On examination, the child is tachypneic with suprasternal and intercostal retractions and nasal flaring, which requires immediate ventilatory support. Lung exam reveals bilateral wheezing and inspiratory crackles. White blood count and differential are normal. CXR is shown in Fig. 83.

155. A correct statement regarding this infection is
a. Outbreaks occur in summer.
b. Most serious infections occur in adults.
c. The spread and mode of transmission is self-inoculation and fomites.
d. It is caused by a double-stranded DNA virus.

156. The treatment of choice in this case would be
a. Steroids
b. Bronchodilator therapy
c. Fluid restriction
d. Aerosolized ribavarin

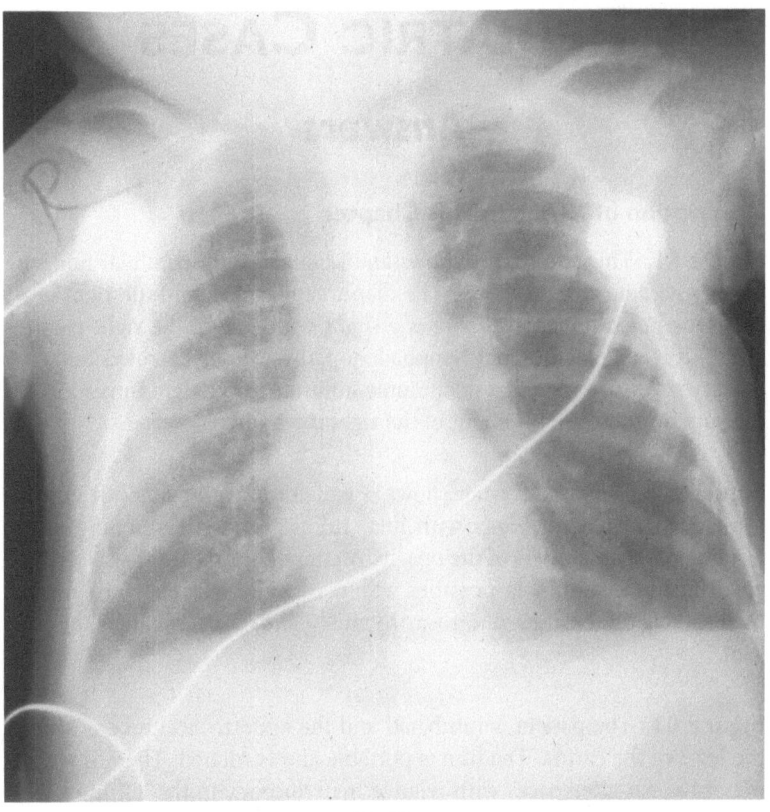

Fig. 83

PEDIATRIC CASES

Answers

Description of X-rays in This Chapter

Figure 81. This chest x-ray shows an ill-defined right parahilar midzone opacity with air bronchogram. The diaphragm is clear and the right heart border is not silhouetted. There is a slight widening of the right paratracheal area, and mediastinal lymphadenopathy cannot be ruled out. The opacity is consistent with a pneumonic infiltrate in the right upper lobe or the superior posterior segment of the right lower lobe.

Figure 82. This chest x-ray shows a widening of the superior and infravascular mediastinal area with hilar fullness and straightening of the AP window. The borders of the opacity on the right side are clearly defined and the mediastinum is possibly widened but consistent with normal mediastinal dimensions due to a thymus gland. This is called the "sail sign."

Figure 83. The patient is intubated and the endotracheal tube is seen at the level of the carina. The film is portable and is rotated. There is widening of the rib interspaces with relative hyperlucency in the left lung. This suggests gas/air trapping and is consistent with bronchiolitis.

General Discussion

The plain chest radiograph in children is very dependent on proper technique. Immobility of the child is crucial, and in a young infant an AP film is often preferred. The difference in cardiothoracic ratio seen in adults in the AP and PA projections is not evident in a child less than 4 years of age. Inspiratory and expiratory views are helpful in evaluating the presence of partially obstructed endobronchial lesions or foreign body. Decubitus films with the downward lung acting as a forced expiratory film may also be helpful in this regard.

Specific Discussion

151–152. The answers are 151-c, 152-a. With a family history of tuberculosis in a close household contact, the likelihood of the patient's illness being active primary TB is very high. Thirty percent of persons with a close contact with active disease have a positive PPD, and this is increased in children under the age of 4 years. About 5% of persons with recent contact may develop active disease. Most children infected with *Mycobacterium tuberculosis* are asymptomatic and their chest x-rays may be normal on initial examination. The most common radiographic presentations in children include hilar and mediastinal lymphadenopathy, segmental lobar infiltrates with consolidation, or pleural effusion or miliary TB. Extrapulmonary tuberculosis occurs in approximately 20% of infants and children with TB. Early involvement may include bone and miliary TB, but later manifestations may include mastoiditis, otorrhea, or pyrexia of chronic duration.

153–154. The answers are 153-b, 154-b. The thymus is composed of two lobes, which are frequently asymmetrical. With increasing age it atrophies and is replaced by fat with streaky or nodular densities. Cystic transformation can occur along the developmental pathway of the thymopharyngeal duct, and in patients with Hodgkin's lymphoma, persistence of these cysts can be seen due to thymic involution. These cysts can persist or even enlarge after radiation treatment or chemotherapy. Rebound thymic hyperplasia is seen in children, where a period of stress associated with thymic involution is followed by regrowth or overgrowth of the gland. However, despite an abnormal increase, the gland maintains its normal arrowhead configuration. Thymomas are neoplasms of the thymic epithelial cells with cystic degeneration and calcification. They are seen in adults, usually in the fifth decade of life. About 40% of adults with thymomas have myasthenia gravis and 15% of patients with myasthenia gravis have thymoma. Thymoma may be associated with hypogammaglobulinemia, red cell aplasia, thyroid carcinoma, or inflammatory bowel disease. Thymic carcinoma is rare but has a poor prognosis due to local and distant metastases. (Refer to Chap. 14 also).

155–156. The answers are 155-c, 156-d. This infant with an upper respiratory infection and signs of respiratory distress has acute bronchiolitis, most likely due to respiratory syncytial virus in this age group. The treatment of choice is aerosolized ribavirin. The chest x-ray shows air trapping. Respiratory syncytial virus is a single-strand RNA virus that spreads through self-inoculation with fomites. Outbreaks occur in winter and spring, and most serious infections occur in the first 2 years of life.

LUNG TRANSPLANT PATIENTS

DIRECTIONS: Each item below contains a question or incomplete statement followed by suggested responses. Select the **one best** response to each question.

Items 157–158

A 32-year-old male underwent a lung transplant 1 year ago. Initially, he had an episode of acute rejection requiring increased immunosuppression. He now presents with symptoms of low-grade fever and generalized fatigue, fever, and weight loss. Chest x-rays (Fig. 84) are obtained.

157. The most likely diagnosis of this patient is

a. Posttransplant lymphomatoid disorder (PTLD)
b. Squamous cell carcinoma
c. Aspergilloma
d. Phantom tumor or pseudotumor

158. The next management step should be

a. Diurectic therapy
b. Amphotericin
c. Needle biopsy
d. Antibiotics

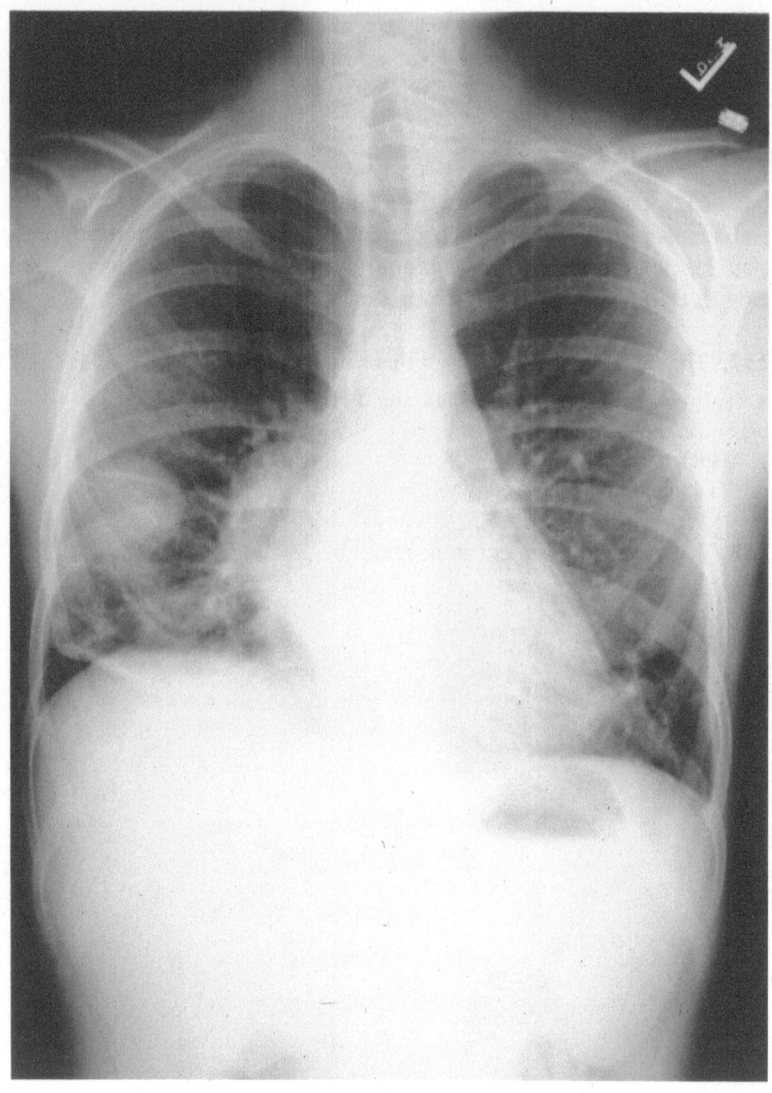

Fig. 84a

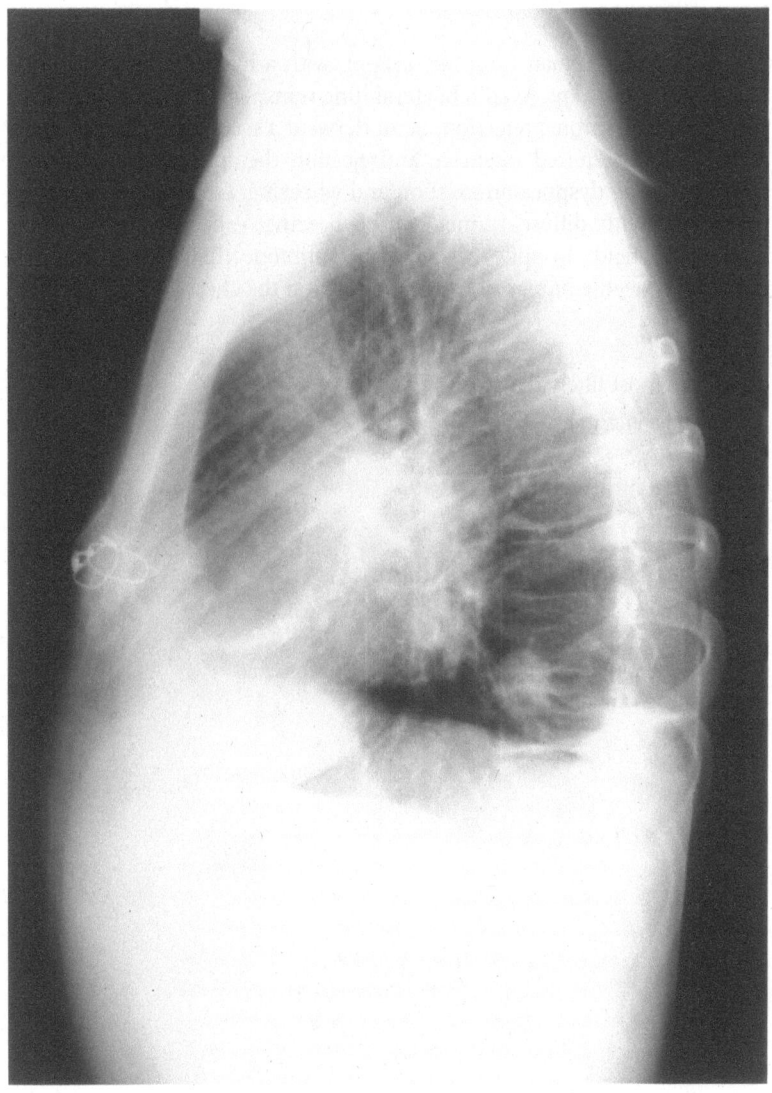

Fig. 84b

Items 159–160

A 25-year-old man from Mississippi, with a history of cystic fibrosis diagnosed at birth, received a bilateral lung transplant 3 years ago. Due to posttransplant chronic rejection, he underwent a second lung transplant 1 year ago and required intensive antirejection therapy. He now presents with worsening dyspnea on exertion and wheezing. On examination, he is tachypneic with diffuse rhonchi and wheezing, especially in the right upper lung field. In spite of empirical antibiotic therapy, he does not improve. A needle biopsy of the lesion seen on the chest x-ray (Fig. 85) is done.

159. The most likely diagnosis is
a. Nocardia infection
b. Blastomycosis
c. Cytomegalovirus infection
d. Aspergillosis

160. The treatment of choice in this case is
a. Stopping antirejection drugs
b. Starting amphotericin
c. Stopping antirejection drugs and starting itraconazole
d. Starting gancycolvir

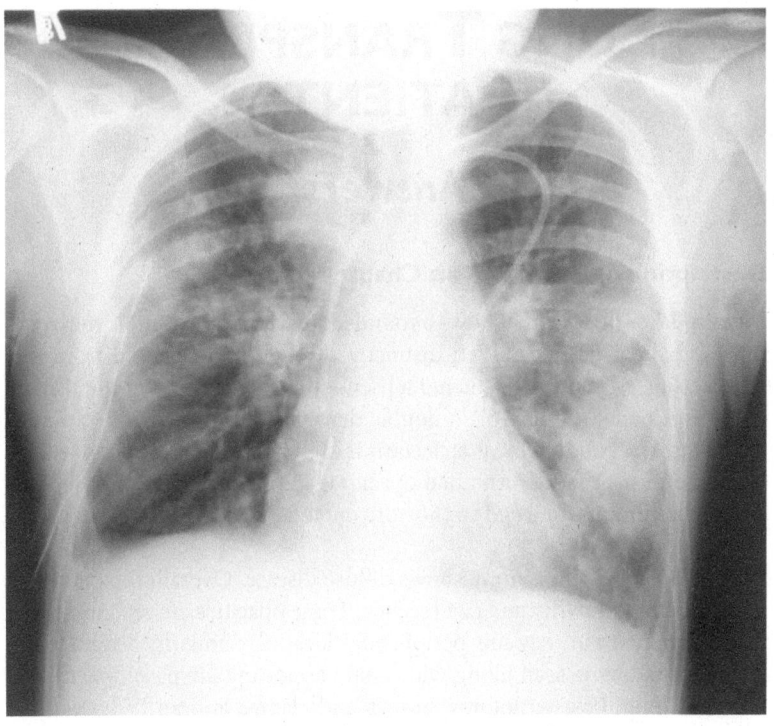

Fig. 85

LUNG TRANSPLANT PATIENTS

Answers

Description of X-rays in This Chapter

Figure 84. The PA view shows a rounded opacity in the right lower zone. The horizontal fissure is seen distinctly through and separate from this opacity, suggesting that this is not a pseudotumor, i.e., fluid in the fissure. (Refer to Chap. 12, Fig. 46.) A double density shadow is seen in the subcarinal area. A band of linear atelectasis is seen in the right lower zone. The lateral confirms that the rounded opacity is in the hilar area and the middle mediastinum, unrelated to the horizontal fissure.

Figure 85. This chest x-ray shows diffuse disease. Overall, the pattern is of confluent nodularity and coalescence. These opacities are seen in the left lower zone, where they are peripherally located. Similarly, a right paratracheal shadow is seen along with cystic-appearing airspace opacities in the right lung. Poststernotomy sutures and clamps and an IV access line leading to the PA are also noted. A small pneumothorax is present on the right side, with a chest tube along the right lateral chest wall.

General Discussion

Lung transplantations are performed primarily for the treatment of pulmonary fibrosis, primary pulmonary hypertension, cystic fibrosis, and end-stage emphysema. Bilateral lung transplantation is preferred in young patients or in cystic fibrosis, where there is an increased risk of donor lung infection from the native lung. Five-year survival is about 50% to 60%. Immediate causes of morbidity and mortality include reperfusion injury, airway injury and ischemia, acute rejection, and infection. Acute rejection is graded by the severity of perivascular infiltration, ranging from minimal to severe. Acute rejection can occur due to subtherapeutic cyclosporin level. A CMV mismatch leads to a high risk of CMV infection. Bacterial pneumonia recurs in the perioperative period and presents with pneumonic symptoms and white cell elevation. Late complications include infections, bronchiectasis, and airway stenosis. Causes of death after the initial postoperative and hospital course include chronic rejection, bronchiolitis obliterans, sepsis, and lymphoproliferative disease. The imaging techniques used in evaluating patients with immune-compromised states begin with a chest x-ray. Although these abnormalities are nonspecific, they are helpful in assessment when viewed in conjunction with other clinical data such as the time of development of the changes. Three primary patterns are generally seen. These are a diffuse interstitial pattern, nodular opacities, and areas of consolidation. Cavitary opacities are seen in necrotizing infections such as those caused by anaerobes and aspergillus. Radiographically, nodular opacities in the transplant patient are due to aspergillus, rhodococcus, posttransplantation lymphoproliferative disorder (PTLD), or CMV infection.

Specific Discussion

157–158. The answers are 157-a, 158-c. The patient has posttransplantation lymphoproliferative disorder (PTLD) confirmed by a needle biopsy. The incidence of PTLD in lung transplant recipients is approximately 2% to 5% and is higher than in other solid organ transplants. It is closely associated with Epstein-Barr virus infection, and children are more prone to develop this disorder. The majority of PTLDs are non-Hodgkin's lymphomas and B-cell tumors. Typical radiographic features include multiple nodules, mediastinal adenopathy, airspace disease, and pleural effusions. Aspergilloma or mycetoma is a fungus ball that occurs in cystic or cavitary disease and is unrelated to lung transplant. Pseudotumor or fluid in the horizontal or oblique fissure occurs in cases of congestive heart failure and is seen radiographically within the confines of these fissures.

159–160. The answers are 159-d, 160-b. Posttransplant infection is the leading cause of mortality following lung transplant. Immunosuppression increases the risk of infection. The transplanted lung is more susceptible than the native lung due to impaired lymphatic drainage, decreased mucociliary clearance, and ischemic injury. Radiographic manifestations may be nonspecific. Bacterial and viral infections occur within the first few months and can present with cough, fever, malaise, and hypoxemia. Psuedomonas, staphylococci, and CMV are characteristically implicated. Fungal infections are less common but are associated with higher mortality. Invasive aspergillosis manifests as pneumonia with airspace consolidation. This patient had signs of airway and airspace disease, and, given his history of intense immunosuppression, aspergillus infection is the most likely cause.

GLOSSARY*

Acinar pattern. A collection of round, patchy, or confluent opacities producing an inhomogeneous shadow, representing one or more anatomic acinar structures rendered opaque by consolidation. The acinus is a portion of lung parenchyma that is distal to the terminal bronchiole and consists of the respiratory bronchiole, alveolar sacs, and alveoli.

Air bronchiologram. A peripherally located air bronchogram. Air is seen in a bronchus, implying a patent airway.

Air bronchogram. A shadow of an air-containing bronchus peripheral to the hilum and surrounded by airless consolidation.

Air-fluid level. A collection of gas and liquid that, when traversed by a horizontal x-ray beam, creates a shadow characterized by a sharp horizontal interface between the gas density above and the liquid density below.

Airspace disease. This includes the gas-containing portion of the lung parenchyma, including the acini, but excludes the interstitial and the conductive portions of the lung. Used synonymously with acinar or alveolar consolidation.

Aorta-pulmonary window. A mediastinal space bounded anteriorly by the posterior surface of the ascending aorta; posteriorly by the anterior surface of the descending aorta; superiorly by the inferior surface of the aortic arch; inferiorly by the superior surface of the left pulmonary artery; medially by the left side of the trachea, the left main bronchus, and the esophagus; and laterally by the left lung. Within it are situated fat, the ductus ligament, the left recurrent laryngeal nerve, and lymph nodes. On a PA view, it appears like the concavity of the numeral 3, with the upper portion of the 3 representing the aorta and the lower portion representing the pulmonary artery. Fullness in this area or obliteration of the space generally represents lymph nodes or masses in that area.

---

*Modified and adapted from Fraser RG et al: *Diagnosis of Diseases of the Chest*, 4th ed. Philadelphia, Saunders, 1999.

Atelectasis. Lesser than normal inflation of all or portion of the lung, i.e., airless segment or lobe, with corresponding loss of volume. Used synonymously with collapse.

Batwing distribution. Also called a butterfly distribution, it is seen on the frontal x-ray and bears a resemblance to a bat in flight, and is said to be due to coalescence of ill-defined parahilar symmetrical opacities.

Bleb. A gas-containing space within or contiguous to the visceral pleura of the lung. It is seen as a thin-walled lucency usually present at the lung apex.

Bulla. A sharply demarcated region of gas-containing space with ruptured alveolar septa and vessels, 1 cm or more in diameter and possessing a wall less than 1 mm thick. Often seen in emphysema.

Carinal angle. The angle formed by the right and left main stem bronchi at the tracheal bifurcation.

Cavity. A mass within the lung parenchyma, the central portion of which has undergone liquefaction necrosis, leaving a gas-containing space with or without fluid. It is present within the lung parenchyma surrounded by a wall whose thickness is greater than 1 mm.

Circumscribed opacity. An opacity that shows a completely or nearly completely visible border.

Coin lesion. A sharply defined small circular opacity within the lung.

Consolidation. Described as a process by which air is replaced by diseased lung as in pneumonia. It contains air bronchograms without volume loss or effacement of the pulmonary vessels.

Cyst. A circumscribed space filled with liquid or gas, whose wall is generally thin and is lined by an epithelium whose thickness is generally greater than 1 mm.

Density. Mass of the substance per unit volume. This term is better replaced by *opacity*.

Diffuse. A term indicating widespread, anatomically contiguous, but not necessarily complete involvement.

Disseminated. A term connoting widespread, anatomically discontinuous involvement.

Doubling time. The time within which a pulmonary nodule or mass will double in volume or increase in diameter by a factor of 1.25.

Fibrocalcific. A term used to define linear or nodular opacities containing calcification, generally seen in the upper lobes and presumed to represent old, granulomatous lesions.

Ground glass pattern. A term designating an extensive, finely granular pattern within which the normal anatomic details are partially obscured, visually like a glass shower door.

Hilum. A specific part of the pulmonary anatomy comprising the shadows at the root of each lung; composed of bronchi, arteries, veins, lymph nodes, nerves, bronchial vessels, and alveolar tissue.

Infiltrate. A nonspecific term implying any substance or cells that occur or spread through the interstitium or alveoli that would be foreign to the lung and accumulate in greater than normal quantity. A better word is *opacity*.

Interstitium. A continuum of loose connective tissue throughout the lung representing the lung between alveolar and capillary basement membrane or the subpleural area between the pleura and the lung, or surrounding the bronchovascular bundles. It is not visible normally, and is seen only when disease or edema increases its volume.

Kerley A lines. Essentially straight, linear opacities 2 to 6 cm in length and 1 to 3 mm in width, usually situated in the upper zone and pointing toward the hilum centrally and directed toward but not extending to the pleural surface peripherally.

Kerley B lines. Straight linear opacities 1.5 to 2 cm in length and 1 to 2 mm in width situated at the lung base and oriented at right angles to the pleural surface.

Kerley C lines. A group of linear opacities producing the appearance of fine net situated at the lung base and representing Kerley B lines en face. These are usually septal lines and a specific feature suggesting lymphatic involvement.

Mass. Any pulmonary or pleural lesion represented on an x-ray with a discrete opacity that is greater than 3 cm in diameter, without regard to its contour, border, or homogeneity.

Miliary pattern. A collection of tiny, discrete opacities in the lung measuring 2 to 4 mm or less in diameter and generally uniform in size and micronodular in pattern.

Nodular pattern. A collection of innumerable small discrete opacities ranging in diameter from 4 to 10 mm, generally uniform in size, widespread in distribution, and without spiculation.

Pneumatocele. A thin-walled, gas-filled space within the lung occurring usually with acute pneumonia (especially staphylococcus) and transient in nature.

Reticular pattern. A collection of innumerable small linear opacities resembling a net that may be fine, medium, or coarse and is associated with pneumoconiosis or interstitial disease.

Silhouette sign. The effacement of the anatomic soft tissue border by either a normal anatomic structure (e.g., the inferior border of the heart and the left diaphragm) or by a pathological state such as the airlessness of adjacent lung and/or accumulation of fluid in the space. It implies loss of the silhouette of the adjacent structure, and therefore an additional abnormal opacity.

Systemic. A term designating involvement of the thoracic structure and tissues as part of a process involving other organs.

Tramline shadows. Slightly convergent linear opacities that suggest tubular structures corresponding to the bronchial tree and represent dilated bronchial walls.

Abbreviations

$A\text{-}aD_{O_2}$	Alveolar-arterial difference of oxygen
ABGs	Arterial blood gases
ACE	Angiotensin converting enzyme
AFB	Acid-fast bacilli
ANA	Antinuclear antibody
ARDS	Adult respiratory distress syndrome
BCG	Bacille Calmette-Guérin (TB vaccine)
BMI	Body mass index
BOOP	Bronchiolitis obliterans with organizing pneumonia
BUN	Blood urea nitrogen
CABG	Coronary artery bypass graft
C-ANCA	Cytoplasmic antineutrophilic cytoplasmic antibody
CAP	Community-acquired pneumonia
COPD	Chronic obstructive pulmonary disease
CPK	Creatine phosphokinase
CT	Computed tomography
CXR	Chest x-ray
DLCO	Diffusing capacity of carbon monoxide
ECG	Electrocardiogram
ESR	Erythrocyte sedimentation rate
FEF_{25-75}	Forced midexpiratory flow rate
FEV_1	Forced expired volume in 1 s
FVC	Forced vital capacity
Hb	Hemoglobin
Hct	Hematocrit
HIV	Human immunodeficiency virus
IgE	Immunoglobulin E
IPF	Idiopathic pulmonary fibrosis
LDH	Lactate dehydrogenase
MRI	Magnetic resonance imaging
NTM	Nontuberculous mycobacteria
PA	Posterior-anterior; pulmonary artery
P_{CO_2}	Partial pressure of carbon dioxide
PCP	*Pneumocystis carinii* pneumonia

PFTs	Pulmonary function tests
P_{O_2}	Partial pressure of oxygen
PPD	Purified protein derivative (TB skin test)
PTH	Parathyroid hormone
RV	Residual volume
SPN	Solitary pulmonary nodule
TLC	Total lung capacity
V/Q	Ventilation/perfusion
WBC	White blood cell

Quick Reference

For each chapter, you will find the appropriate clinical findings and matched radiographic differential diagnoses. Refer to chest x-rays and questions pertaining to them for further elaboration.

Chapter	Clinical Key Word(s) or Hints	Diagnosis	Figures	Questions
1. Solitary Pulmonary Nodule	• Endemic area • Positive PPD • Orthodeoxia • Smoker	• Cocci • Granuloma • AVM • Adenocarcinoma	1–4	1–7
2. Multiple Pulmonary Nodules	• Low-grade fever • Occupational exposure • Weight loss • Pneumonectomy	• Miliary disease • Silicosis • Metastatic disease • Metastatic disease	5–8	8–14
3. Lung Masses	• Abnormal labs • Fever/chills • Retrocardiac opacity	• Carcinoma • Round pneumonia • Carcinoma	9–11	15–18
4. Cavitary Lesions	• Foul-smelling sputum • Nasal discharge; hemoptysis • Old TB; COPD • Hemoptysis • IVDA; night sweats • Weight loss	• Lung abscess • Wegener's granulomatosis • NTM • Aspergilloma • Tuberculosis • Squamous cell CA	12–17	19–29
5. Hyperlucent Lung	• Shortness of breath • Exercise intolerance	• Emphysema • Bulla	18–20	30–35
6. Cysts and Cystic-Appearing Lesions	• Productive cough/SOB • Hx walking pneumonias	• Infected bulla • Bronchiectasis	21–24	36–43

Chapter	Clinical Key Word(s) or Hints	Diagnosis	Figures	Questions
	• Infertility	• Immotile cilia syndrome		
	• Repeated infections	• Sequestration of lung		
	• Cough/repeated infection	• Cystic fibrosis		
7. Diffuse Interstitial Disease	• Clubbing, crackles	• Idiopathic pulmonary fibrosis	25–30	44–55
	• Weakness	• Polymyositis		
	• Shortness of breath	• Sarcoidosis		
	• Shortness of breath	• BOOP		
	• Shortness of breath	• Hypersensitivity pneumonitis		
	• Shortness of breath	• Lymphangitic spread		
8. Diffuse Airspace Disease	• Hemoptysis	• Alveolar hemorrhage	31–34	56–59
	• Increased A-aDo_2	• ARDS		
	• Sputum/non-res infiltrate	• Bronchoalveolar CA		
	• Difficulty swallowing	• Aspiration		
9. Focal Airspace Homogeneous Opacities	• Endobronchial obstruction	• RUL atelectasis	35–38	60–68
	• LLL mass on FOB	• LLL sail sign		
	• Horner syndrome	• Pancoast tumor		
	• Mucus plug	• RUL atelectasis		
10. Focal Airspace Nonhomogeneous Opacities	• Fever, chills	• Multilobar pneumonia	39–42	69–77
	• Fever, chills	• LLL pneumonia		
	• Fever/hx of ETOH	• Klebsiella pneumonia		
	• Flulike illness	• Staphylococcal pneumonia		

Chapter	Clinical Key Word(s) or Hints	Diagnosis	Figures	Questions
11. Unilateral Complete Opacification	• Transmitted sounds • Decreased breath sounds • Stony dullness	• Pneumonectomy • Atelectasis • Pleural effusion	43–45	78–80
12. Pleural Disease	• CHF/SOB • Dullness on percussion • SOB/chest pain • Occupational hx • Old TB • Hx trauma	• Interlobar effusion • Pleural effusion • Pneumothorax • Pleural plaques • Calcified pleura • Hemothorax	46–51	81–90
13. Pulmonary Vascular Disease	• Metallic taste • Acute SOB • Syncope	• HG embolism • Pulmonary embolism • PPH	52–55	91–97
14. Mediastinal Compartments	• Incidental • Muscle weakness • Erythema nodosum • Lightheadedness • Reduced stamina/cough • Uncontrolled HTN • Weakness, dysphagia	• Substernal goiter • Thymoma • Hilar calcification • PA aneurysm • BHL • Aortic aneurysm • CA esophagus	56–62	98–110
15. Cardiac and Pericardial Disease	• Distant heart sounds • Hx myocardial infarction • Summation gallop • Pericardial effusion • Hx TB • Abnormal CVS exam • Abnormal auscultation	• Pericardial effusion • LV aneurysm • CHF • Pneumopericardium • Pericardial calcification • MS with LVF • Atrial septal defect	63–69	111–124

Chapter	Clinical Key Word(s) or Hints	Diagnosis	Figures	Questions
16. Chest Wall and Skeletal Deformities	• HX MVA • SOB/ osteoporosis • Nonspecific discomfort • Hx TB	• Rib fractures • Kyphoscoliosis • Pectus • Thoracoplasty	70–73	125–135
17. Diaphragmatic Lesions	• Postprandial symptoms • Asymptomatic • SOB	• Hiatal hernia • Bochdalek hernia • Diaphragmatic paralysis	74–76	136–140
18. Lines/Devices/ Complications in ICU	• Palpable crunch • Hemoptysis • Sudden shock • Focal decreased breath sounds	• Pneumo- mediastinum • Vascular injury • Pneumothorax • RMS intubation	77–80	141–150
19. Pediatric Cases	• Contact history • Incidental finding • Respiratory distress	• Primary tuberculosis • Thymoma • RSV bronchiolitis	81–83	151–156
20. Lung Transplant Patients	• Immuno- supressed • Wheezing	• Nodular densities • Nodular cavitary opacities	84–85	157–160

SUGGESTED READING

Fraser RG et al: *Diagnosis of the Diseases of the Chest,* 4th ed. Philadelphia, Saunders, 1999.

Freundlich IM, Bragg DG: *A Radiologic Approach to Diseases of the Chest,* 2d ed. Baltimore, Williams & Wilkins, 1997.

Murray JF, Nadel JA: *Textbook of Respiratory Medicine,* 2d ed. Philadelphia, Saunders, 1994.

Slone RM et al: *Thoracic Imaging: A Practical Approach.* New York, McGraw-Hill, 1999.

Notes

Notes

Notes

Notes

Notes

Notes

Notes

Notes

Notes

Notes

Notes